Management of Metatarsalgia and Painful Lesser Toe Deformities

Editor

TODD A. IRWIN

FOOT AND ANKLE CLINICS

www.foot.theclinics.com

Consulting Editor
MARK S. MYERSON

March 2018 • Volume 23 • Number 1

ELSEVIER

1600 John F. Kennedy Boulevard • Suite 1800 • Philadelphia, Pennsylvania, 19103-2899

http://www.theclinics.com

FOOT AND ANKLE CLINICS Volume 23, Number 1
March 2018 ISSN 1083-7515, ISBN-13: 978-0-323-58152-3

Editor: Lauren Boyle
Developmental Editor: Meredith Madeira

Foot and Ankle Clinics (ISSN 1083-7515) is published quarterly by Elsevier, Inc., 360 Park Avenue South, New York, NY 10010-1710. Months of issue are March, June, September, and December. Periodicals postage paid at New York, NY, and additional mailing offices. Subscription price per year is $326.00 (US individuals), $519.00 (US institutions), $100.00 (US students), $367.00 (Canadian individuals), $623.00 (Canadian institutions), $215.00 (Canadian students), $460.00 (international individuals), $623.00 (international institutions), and $215.00 (international students). To receive student/resident rate, orders must be accompanied by name of affiliated institution, date of term, and the *signature* of program/residency coordinator on institution letterhead. Orders will be billed at individual rate until proof of status is received. Foreign air speed delivery is included in all *Clinics* subscription prices. All prices are subject to change without notice. **POSTMASTER:** Send address changes to *Foot and Ankle Clinics*, Elsevier Health Sciences Division, Subscription Customer Service, 3251 Riverport Lane, Maryland Heights, MO 63043. **Customer Service: 1-800-654-2452 (US and Canada). From outside of the United States and Canada, call 314-447-8871. Fax: 314-447-8029. E-mail: JournalsCustomerService-usa@ elsevier.com (for print support); JournalsOnlineSupport-usa@elsevier.com (for online support).**

Reprints. For copies of 100 or more, of articles in this publication, please contact the Commercial Reprints Department, Elsevier Inc., 360 Park Avenue South, New York, NY 10010-1710. Tel.: 212-633-3874; Fax: 212-633-3820; E-mail: reprints@elsevier.com.

Contributors

CONSULTING EDITOR

MARK S. MYERSON, MD
Medical Director, The Foot and Ankle Association, Inc, Baltimore, Maryland, USA

EDITOR

TODD A. IRWIN, MD
OrthoCarolina Foot and Ankle Institute, Associate Professor, Carolinas Medical Center, Charlotte, North Carolina, USA

AUTHORS

SAMUEL B. ADAMS, MD
Assistant Professor, Foot and Ankle Division, Department of Orthopedic Surgery, Duke University Medical Center, Durham, North Carolina, USA

ALEXEJ BARG, MD
Assistant Professor, Department of Orthopedics, The University of Utah, Salt Lake City, Utah, USA

DANIEL BAUMFELD, MD
Adjunct Professor, Federal University of Minas Gerais, Belo Horizonte, Brazil

EZEQUIEL CATA, MD
Department of Orthopaedic Surgery, Sanatorio Allende, Córdoba, Argentina

FERNANDA CATENA, MD
Foot and Ankle Specialist, Orthopaedics and Sports Medecine Department, Hospital Nove de Julho, Sao Paulo, Brazil

ROSE E. CORTINA, MD
Orthopedic Surgery Resident, University of Kansas Medical Center, Kansas City, Kansas, USA

JESSE F. DOTY, MD
Director of Foot and Ankle Surgery, Department of Orthopedic Surgery, Erlanger Health System, Assistant Professor, The University of Tennessee College of Medicine, Chattanooga, Tennessee, USA

ANDREW E. FEDERER, MD
Orthopaedic Surgery Resident, Department of Orthopedic Surgery, Duke University Medical Center, Durham, North Carolina, USA

FRED T. FINNEY, MD
Department of Orthopaedic Surgery, University of Michigan, Ann Arbor, Michigan, USA

JASON A. FOGLEMAN, MD
Department of Orthopedic Surgery, Erlanger Health System, The University of Tennessee College of Medicine, Chattanooga, Tennessee, USA

SOLENNE FREY-OLLIVIER, MD
Centre du Pied, Marseille, France

MARIANNE HÉLIX-GIORDANINO, MD
Centre du Pied, Marseille, France

JAMES R. HOLMES, MD
Assistant Professor, Department of Orthopaedic Surgery, University of Michigan, Ann Arbor, Michigan, USA

RAYMOND Y. HSU, MD
Orthopedic Foot and Ankle Fellow, Department of Orthopedics, The University of Utah, Salt Lake City, Utah, USA

SIMON LEE, MD
Assistant Professor, Department of Orthopedic Surgery, Rush University Medical Center, Chicago, Illinois, USA

BRANDON L. MORRIS, MD
Orthopedic Surgery Resident, University of Kansas Medical Center, Kansas City, Kansas, USA

CAIO NERY, MD
Associate Professor, UNIFESP - Federal University of São Paulo, São Paulo, Brazil

FLORIAN NICKISCH, MD
Associate Professor, Department of Orthopedics, The University of Utah, Salt Lake City, Utah, USA

PHINIT PHISITKUL, MD
Private Practice, Coralville, Iowa, USA

BARBARA PICLET-LEGRÉ, MD
Centre du Pied, Marseille, France

VEERABHADRA "BABU" REDDY, MD
Clinical Assistant Professor, Department of Surgery, Texas A&M Health Science Center College of Medicine, Bryan, Texas, USA; Faculty, Foot and Ankle Surgery Fellowship Program, Baylor University Medical Center at Dallas, Dallas, Texas, USA

DAVID REDFERN, FRCS (Tr&Orth)
Consultant Orthopaedic Surgeon, London Foot and Ankle Centre, Hospital of St John & St Elizabeth, London, United Kingdom

KARL M. SCHWEITZER Jr, MD
Assistant Professor, Foot and Ankle Division, Department of Orthopedic Surgery, Duke University Medical Center, Durham, North Carolina, USA

JEFFREY D. SEYBOLD, MD
Twin Cities Orthopedics, Edina, Minnesota, USA

DAVID M. TAINTER, MD
Orthopaedic Surgery Resident, Department of Orthopedic Surgery, Duke University Medical Center, Durham, North Carolina, USA

PAUL G. TALUSAN, MD
Assistant Professor, Department of Orthopaedic Surgery, University of Michigan, Ann Arbor, Michigan, USA

EMILY C. VAFEK, MD
Fellow, Department of Orthopedic Surgery, Rush University Medical Center, Chicago, Illinois, USA

BRYAN G. VOPAT, MD
Assistant Professor of Orthopedic Surgery, University of Kansas Medical Center, Kansas City, Kansas, USA

JACOB R. ZIDE, MD
Department of Orthopaedic Surgery, Baylor University Medical Center, Dallas, Texas, USA

Editorial Advisory Board

Contents

Preface: Management of Metatarsalgia and Lesser Toe Deformities xv

Todd A. Irwin

Anatomy and Physiology of the Lesser Metatarsophalangeal Joints 1

Fred T. Finney, Ezequiel Cata, James R. Holmes, and Paul G. Talusan

Knowledge and command of anatomy is paramount to effectively treating disorders of the lesser metatarsophalangeal (MTP) joints. The osseous structures consist of the proximal phalanx of the toe and the metatarsal head. The soft tissues on the dorsum of the MTP joint include the joint capsule and the tendons of extensor digitorum longus and extensor digitorum brevis. The proper and accessory collateral ligaments form the medial and lateral walls and contribute to stability in the coronal and sagittal planes. The plantar plate forms the plantar border of the MTP joint and stabilizes the MTP joint against hyperextension and dorsal translation.

Conservative Management of Metatarsalgia and Lesser Toe Deformities 9

Andrew E. Federer, David M. Tainter, Samuel B. Adams, and
Karl M. Schweitzer Jr

There are several forefoot conditions that can result in metatarsal head pain. Various points of the gait cycle can predispose the metatarsal heads to pain based on intrinsic and extrinsic imbalances. Metatarsalgia can further be classified according to primary, secondary, or iatrogenic etiologies. Within these groups, conservative management is the first line of treatment and can often obviate surgical intervention. Depending on the cause of pain, proper shoewear, orthoses, and inserts coupled with targeted physical therapy can alleviate most symptoms of metatarsalgia and lesser toe deformities.

Treatment of Metatarsalgia with Distal Osteotomies 21

David Redfern

Many different distal metatarsal osteotomies have been described in the surgical treatment of metatarsalgia. The surgeon should use such osteotomies judiciously, and indeed, in the author's experience, they are infrequently required and are certainly not a first port of call. In cases in which nonoperative treatments have failed, a thorough understanding of the causes of metatarsalgia and a detailed clinical assessment of the patient are essential if good surgical outcomes are to be achieved. If using distal metatarsal osteotomies as part of the surgical plan, then the author favors extraarticular percutaneous osteotomies to minimize postoperative stiffness.

Treatment of Metatarsalgia with Proximal Osteotomies 35

Emily C. Vafek and Simon Lee

Metatarsalgia is among the most common sources of forefoot pain. Proximal metatarsal osteotomies are an important technique in the armamentarium of the surgeon treating metatarsalgia that has failed nonoperative management. Proximal osteotomies can provide powerful deformity correction with precise control to both shorten and elevate the metatarsal head. However, they can be technically challenging, difficult to attain satisfactory fixation, require increased postoperative immobilization, and can result in transfer lesions. There are numerous described techniques with little supporting evidence, and more research is needed to establish the optimal procedure to reliably alleviate patient's symptoms while minimizing complications.

Metatarsal Osteotomies: Complications   47

Veerabhadra "Babu" Reddy

Metatarsal osteotomies can be divided into proximal and distal. The proximal osteotomies, such as the oblique, segmental, set cut, and Barouk-Rippstein-Toullec osteotomy, all provide the ability to significantly change the position of the metatarsal head without violating the joint. These osteotomies, however, have a high rate of nonunion when done without internal fixation and can lead to transfer metatarsalgia when done without regard to the parabola of metatarsal head position. Distal osteotomies such as the Weil and Helal offer superior healing but have an increased incidence of recurrent metatarsalgia, joint stiffness, and floating toe.

Gastrocnemius Recession for Metatarsalgia   57

Rose E. Cortina, Brandon L. Morris, and Bryan G. Vopat

Metatarsalgia is a common cause of plantar forefoot pain. Causes of metatarsalgia include foot anatomy, gait mechanics, and foot and ankle deformity. One specific cause, mechanical metatarsalgia, occurs because of gastrocnemius muscle contracture, which overloads the forefoot. Muscular imbalance of the gastrocnemius complex alters gait mechanics, which increases recruitment of the toe extensor musculature, thereby altering forefoot pressure. Patients with concomitant metatarsalgia and gastrocnemius contracture demonstrate ankle equinus and a positive Silfverskiold test. Nonoperative therapeutic modalities are mainstays of treatment. In patients in whom these treatments fail to provide metatarsalgia symptomatic relief, gastrocnemius muscle lengthening is a therapeutic option.

Treatment of Flexible Lesser Toe Deformities   69

Solenne Frey-Ollivier, Fernanda Catena, Marianne Hélix-Giordanino, and Barbara Piclet-Legré

Lesser toe deformities are among the most common complaints presented to foot and ankle specialists. These deformities present in variable ways, which makes surgical decision making complex. For every type of deformity, there could be a combination of soft tissues and bony procedures, chosen according to the surgeon's preferences. This article first describes the modern classification of lesser toe deformities and then presents the different treatments and procedures available for those flexible deformities. In addition, this article proposes an algorithm based on clinical/radiologic evaluation and step-by-step surgical decision making.

Treatment of Rigid Hammer-Toe Deformity: Permanent Versus Removable Implant Selection **91**

Jesse F. Doty and Jason A. Fogleman

Hammer-toe deformities that fail nonoperative treatment can be successfully addressed with proximal interphalangeal joint resection arthroplasty or fusion. The goal of surgery is to eliminate the deformity and rigidly fix the toe in a well-aligned position. Hammer-toe correction procedures can be performed with temporary Kirschner wire (K-wire) fixation for 3 to 6 weeks with high success rates. Pain relief with successful hammer-toe correction approaches 90%; patient satisfaction rates approximate 84%. Although complication rates are rare in most series, there remains a concern regarding exposed temporary K-wire fixation, which has led to the development of multiple permanent internal fixation options.

Lesser Metatarsophalangeal Joint Instability: Treatment with Tendon Transfers **103**

Caio Nery and Daniel Baumfeld

Complex digital deformities and metatarsophalangeal joint instability encompass a wide range of pathology, and one must identify the different degrees of ligamentous disruption. It is important to address a combination of procedures to treat gross deformities of the lesser toes. Surgical treatment should be individualized and requires a sequential process for adequate reduction and deformity correction. There is no gold standard procedure for every deformity. Although residual stiffness can result from tendon transfer, overall patient satisfaction levels remain high when it is performed under the proper indications and concomitantly with other procedures to gain full correction of these challenging deformities.

Lesser Metatarsophalangeal Joint Instability: Advancements in Plantar Plate Reconstruction **127**

Raymond Y. Hsu, Alexej Barg, and Florian Nickisch

The plantar plate and associated collateral ligaments are the main stabilizers of each of the lesser metatarsophalangeal joints. Although clinical examination and plain radiographs are usually sufficient to establish the diagnosis of a plantar plate tear, MRI or fluoroscopic arthrograms may help in specific cases. Recent results with a dorsal approach to plantar plate repair are promising with respect to pain relief and patient satisfaction.

Managing Complications of Lesser Toe and Metatarsophalangeal Joint Surgery **145**

Phinit Phisitkul

The anatomy of the lesser toes is highly complicated and not yet well understood. The high propensity of the metatarsophalangeal joint to develop hyperextension deformity should be recognized. Surgeons should provide each patient with a realistic expectation for lesser toe reconstructive procedures. A successful surgical result requires a well-planned procedure, accurate execution using proper techniques, and meticulous postoperative care. When complications occur, surgeons should identify culprits so that proper treatment strategies can be successfully executed. This article discusses a wide array of tactics to manage common complications in lesser toe surgery.

Treatment of Freiberg Disease   **157**

Jeffrey D. Seybold and Jacob R. Zide

> Freiberg disease, or osteochondrosis of the lesser metatarsal head, usually involves the second metatarsal and presents during the second or third decade of life. Conservative measures to relieve pressure on the affected metatarsal head are the first-line treatments, with good success for Smillie stage I to III disease. Operative treatments are divided into joint-preserving and joint-reconstructing procedures. Although multiple case series describe success with numerous techniques, there are no established guidelines for treatment. All surgical techniques carry a risk of a stiff or floating toe and transfer metatarsalgia. This article reviews the current surgical treatment options for Freiberg disease.

FOOT AND ANKLE CLINICS

FORTHCOMING ISSUES

June 2018
Hallux Valgus Deformity and Treatment:
A Three-Dimensional Approach
Woo-Chun Lee, *Editor*

September 2018
The Subtalar Joint
Norman Espinosa, *Editor*

December 2018
Managing Instabilities of the Foot and Ankle
Andrea Veljkovic, *Editor*

RECENT ISSUES

December 2017
Treatment of Acute and Chronic Tendon
Rupture and Tendinopathy
Selene Parekh, *Editor*

September 2017
The Flatfoot: What Goes Wrong with
Treatment
Kent Ellington, *Editor*

June 2017
Current Updates in Total Ankle Arthroplasty
J. Chris Coetzee, *Editor*

RELATED INTEREST

Podiatric Clinics of North America, January 2017 (Vol. 34, No. 1)
The Diabetic Charcot Foot and Ankle: A Multidisciplinary Team Approach
Thomas Zgonis, *Editor*

THE CLINICS ARE NOW AVAILABLE ONLINE!
Access your subscription at:
www.theclinics.com

Preface

Management of Metatarsalgia and Lesser Toe Deformities

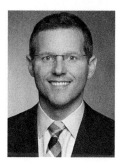

Todd A. Irwin, MD
Editor

The forefoot, and in particular, the lesser toes, can present challenging problems for both patients and surgeons alike. As a frequent source of pain and dysfunction, patients seek solutions for the discomfort, deformity, and shoe-wear issues that go along with forefoot problems. These solutions range from simple offloading inserts to complex reconstructive surgery. As with most orthopedic issues, careful diagnostic evaluation is critical for accurate diagnosis and appropriate treatment.

This issue of *Foot and Ankle Clinics of North America* provides an excellent overview of the current state of treating metatarsalgia and lesser toe deformities. The past several years have seen new advancements in surgical philosophy and technique for these difficult problems. From less invasive surgery to implant type to a renewed interest in anatomic reconstruction, particularly of the lesser metatarsophalangeal joint, multiple treatment options are discussed. I often find myself advising patients that the lesser toes sometimes "have a mind of their own," thereby alluding to the unpredictable nature of lesser toe surgery. As such, it seemed pertinent to dedicate time reviewing the complications seen treating these challenging problems. It is hoped that this issue will be able to provide the reader with a new level of comprehension, or potentially inspire novel research and techniques to take our craft to the next level.

Foot Ankle Clin N Am 23 (2018) xv–xvi
https://doi.org/10.1016/j.fcl.2017.10.003
1083-7515/18/© 2017 Published by Elsevier Inc.

foot.theclinics.com

I would like to thank this expert panel of surgeons for their contributions and for providing excellent insight. I would also like to thank Dr Myerson for the opportunity to be guest editor of this issue, as I have found *Foot and Ankle Clinics of North America* to be an outstanding resource during my career.

Todd A. Irwin, MD
OrthoCarolina Foot and Ankle Institute
Carolinas Medical Center
2001 Vail Avenue, Suite 200B
Charlotte, NC 28207, USA

E-mail address:
todd.irwin@orthocarolina.com

Anatomy and Physiology of the Lesser Metatarsophalangeal Joints

Fred T. Finney, MD[a], Ezequiel Cata, MD[b], James R. Holmes, MD[a], Paul G. Talusan, MD[a],*

KEYWORDS

- Plantar plate • MTP joint • Collateral ligaments • Metatarsalgia

KEY POINTS

- The osseous structures that make up the lesser metatarsophalangeal joints are the proximal phalanx of the toe and the metatarsal head.
- Because of the shape of the articulating surfaces, the metatarsophalangeal joint is unstable.
- The flexor digitorum longus, flexor digitorum brevis, extensor digitorum longus, extensor digitorum brevis, and the intrinsic muscles of the foot provide active motion at the metatarsophalangeal joints.
- The static stabilizers of the metatarsophalangeal joints are the plantar plate, collateral ligaments, deep transverse intermetatarsal ligament, and the joint capsule.

INTRODUCTION

Knowledge and command of anatomy is paramount to effectively treating disorders of the musculoskeletal system. Despite a multitude of clinical problems and surgical solutions related to the forefoot, anatomic studies of the lesser metatarsophalangeal (MTP) joints are somewhat limited when compared with other regions of the body.

The osseous structures that provide the skeletal framework for the MTP joint consists of the proximal phalanx of the toe and the metatarsal head. The soft tissues on the dorsum of the MTP joint include the joint capsule and the tendons of extensor digitorum longus (EDL) and extensor digitorum brevis (EDB). The proper and accessory collateral ligaments form the medial and lateral walls, and the plantar plate forms the plantar border of the MTP joint. The flexor digitorum longus (FDL) and flexor digitorum brevis (FDB) tendons lie on the plantar surface of the plantar plate.

Disclosure Statement: Talusan, Holmes, and Finney are recipients of a research grant related to plantar plate repair from Paragon 28.
[a] Department of Orthopaedic Surgery, University of Michigan, 2098 South Main Street, Ann Arbor, MI 48103, USA; [b] Department of Orthopaedic Surgery, Sanatorio Allende, Independencia 757, Cordoba Capital, Córdoba, Argentina
* Corresponding author.
E-mail address: ptalusan@med.umich.edu

Foot Ankle Clin N Am 23 (2018) 1–7
https://doi.org/10.1016/j.fcl.2017.09.002
1083-7515/18/© 2017 Elsevier Inc. All rights reserved.

foot.theclinics.com

Nery and colleagues[1] described the lesser MTP joint anatomy from an intra-articular, arthroscopic perspective. The medial and lateral gutters contain the medial and lateral dome of metatarsal head, inferior corners of proximal phalanx, accessory collateral ligaments, proper collateral ligaments, and the medial and lateral portions of plantar plate. The central portion consists of the central dome of the metatarsal head, concavity of the proximal phalanx articular surface, the insertion of the plantar plate into the base of the proximal phalanx, a central synovial V-shaped recess between the medial and lateral bundles of the plantar plate insertion, and the central proximal phalanx.[1] The plantar plate forms the floor of the MTP joint and it is a firm fibrocartilage rectangular structure and is considered to be the most important stabilizer of MTP joint.

The purpose of these anatomic structures is to provide stability and mobility to the MTP joint, especially during load-bearing activities. The flexor, extensor, and intrinsic muscles of the foot power movement at the MTP joint but may also act as dynamic stabilizers. Most of the attention in the recent literature has focused on examining the static stabilizers, such as the plantar plate and collateral ligaments.

OSTEOLOGY

The MTP joints are synovial joints with an elliptical articular surface.[2] The distal artic-ular surface of the metatarsal head is bicondylar, with two plantar articular sections separated by a concavity in the center. The lateral condyle is typically larger than the medial condyle.[3] The convex metatarsal heads articulate with the shallow concave base of the proximal phalanx. This "glenoid" cavity is smaller than the articular surface of the metatarsal head creating a somewhat unstable articulation at the MTP joint.[3] The epicondyles on the medial and lateral surface of the metatarsal heads are the origin for the fan-shaped proper and accessory collateral ligaments (**Fig. 1A**).[3]

The foot has long been considered to function as a tripod with the "triangle of sup-port" formed by the first metatarsal head, the fifth metatarsal head, and the calcaneal tuberosity.[4] A multitude of hindfoot and midfoot deformities and injuries can alter the tripod of the foot and affect the relative lengths of the lesser metatarsals in relation to the first and fifth metatarsals.[5] Also, long lesser metatarsals may interrupt the "triangle of support" and lead to painful conditions.[6,7] It is difficult to quantify relative metatarsal length clinically, and various authors have described radiologic methods of measuring relative metatarsal length.[8]

Some authors have challenged the dogma of the "triangle of support" and the as-sociation of long metatarsals and lesser MTP joint problems.[9–11] One such study used a pressure-sensing device to measure plantar pressures during midstance of the gait cycle in asymptomatic volunteers.[10] They found that at midstance, the highest mean pressures were located beneath the second and third metatarsal heads, fol-lowed by the heel and fourth and fifth metatarsal heads, and the least amount of pres-sure was beneath the first metatarsal head.[10]

Menz and colleagues[9] reported on the relative length of the metatarsals in patients with and without forefoot pain and found that patients with forefoot pain had increased plantar pressures beneath the lesser metatarsal heads, but did not have significantly longer metatarsals than asymptomatic patients.

A study that supports the "triangle of support" but argues against the significance of relative metatarsal length was performed by Kaipel and colleagues.[11] Pedobarogra-phy and radiographs were performed in a group of patients with callosities beneath a lesser metatarsal head and an asymptomatic control group. They found that there was no difference in relative metatarsal length in patients with and without

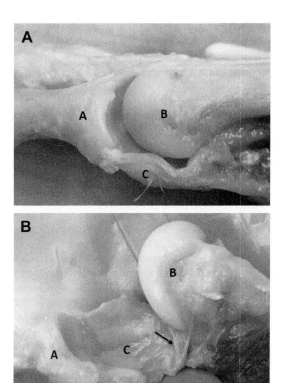

Fig. 1. (*A*) Sagittal view of lesser MTP joint. (*B*) Sagittal view of lesser MTP joint with collaterals removed and joint dislocated: A, proximal phalanx; B, metatarsal head; C, plantar plate with collateral ligaments transected. Synovial-like proximal attachment to the metatarsal neck indicated by arrow.

metatarsalgia. However, they did report that patients with metatarsalgia demonstrated decreased maximal force beneath the first metatarsal head.[11]

PLANTAR PLATE

On the plantar aspect of the lesser MTP joints lies the plantar plate. It is a thick, trapezoidal structure that consists of fibrocartilage[12] and type I collagen that is similar to the composition of the knee meniscus and annulus fibrosis of the intervertebral disc.[13] The plantar plate is the primary static stabilizer to dorsal translation and hyperextension of the proximal phalanx,[1,14] although the collateral ligaments also play an important role in sagittal plane stability.[14]

Distally, the plantar plate inserts firmly to the plantar base of the proximal phalanx.[1,13] Nery and colleagues[1] described a medial and lateral bundle at the insertion into the proximal phalanx separated by a small synovial recess. The proximal portion of the plantar plate originates from the flare of the plantar surface of the metatarsal neck with a loose and fragile synovial appearance (**Fig. 1**B).[1,15]

Several soft tissue structures insert onto the plantar plate on the medial and lateral sides and proximally. The proximal portion of the plantar plate has an attachment to the distal aspect of the plantar fascia, which is its most substantial distal insertion.[1,12,16] The deep transverse metatarsal ligament (DTML) and the collateral ligaments attach to the medial and lateral borders of the plantar plate.[1,13,15] The plantar surface of the plantar plate is smooth and grooved to provide a gliding surface for the flexor tendons and the flexor tendon sheath is invested into the medial and lateral borders of the plantar plate.[13,15]

The organization of the collagen bundles in the plantar plate suggests that it is designed to withstand compressive and tensile forces.[12,17] In a histologic study, Gregg and colleagues[17] observed that the central collagen bundles largely run longitudinally and peripherally, the collagen bundles run largely transversely and merge with collateral ligaments and DTML.

PROPER AND ACCESSORY COLLATERAL LIGAMENTS

The collateral ligaments originate on the medial and lateral epicondyles of the lesser metatarsals and form the walls of the MTP joint.[1] They are made up of two distinct bundles: the proper collateral ligament and the accessory collateral ligament.[12] The proper collateral ligament lies dorsal to the accessory collateral ligament. It is fusiform in shape and courses obliquely to insert on the medial and lateral tubercles of the proximal phalanx.[1,12] The accessory collateral ligament is broad and fan-shaped and inserts broadly along the medial and lateral border of the plantar plate (**Fig. 2**).[3,12]

The main function of the collateral ligaments is to stabilize the joint in the transverse plane[3,12,18] but they also have a significant contribution as a restraint against dorsal translation and hyperextension of the proximal phalanx at the MTP joint.[14,19,20]

EXTENSOR TENDONS

The extensors of the MTP joint are the EDL and EDB.[21,22] The EDL trifurcates at the level of the proximal phalanx to form a medial, central, and lateral slip.[21,22] The central slip inserts onto the base of middle phalanx and the medial and lateral slips travel distally and converge as the terminal tendon, which inserts on the base of distal phalanx.[21,22] The EDB tendon runs obliquely and lateral to the EDL tendon at the level of the midfoot, and the tendons converge to form a single extensor apparatus more distally, just proximal to the trifurcation (**Fig. 3**).[21,22]

The extensor sling stabilizes the extensor tendons, similar to the sagittal bands of the hand extensors, and it is a fibroaponeurotic structure at the level of the MTP joint with transversely oriented fibers. It covers the EDB and EDL tendons and continues plantarly to insert on the plantar plate, DTML, and the sheath of the FDL and FDP tendons.[22]

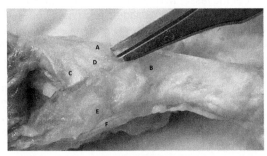

Fig. 2. Sagittal view of lesser MTP joint: A, metatarsal head; B, proximal phalanx; C, accessory collateral ligament; D, proper collateral ligament; E, plantar plate; F, flexor tendons.

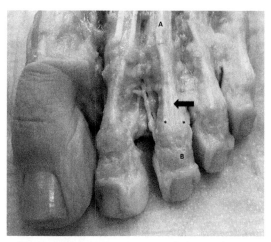

Fig. 3. Dorsal view of lesser MTP joints. A, extensor digitorum longus tendon. The tendon trifurcates at the level of the MTP joint into the middle slip (*arrow*) and the medial and lateral slips (*asterisks*). The medial and lateral slips converge to become the terminal tendon (B) and insert into the distal phalanx.

LUMBRICALS AND INTEROSSEI

The dorsal and plantar interossei and the tendons of the lumbricals insert onto the base of the proximal phalanx and act to flex the lesser MTP joints.[3] The dorsal interossei are located laterally and the plantar interossei are on the medial side.[1,15] The interossei tendons travel on sides of MTP joint and pass dorsal to the DTML.[13,15] They then pass through a tunnel between extensor sling and joint capsule and blend with the dorsal aponeurosis to act as extensors of the interphalangeal joints.[21] The interossei also have some fibers that insert onto the plantar plate.[15] The lumbricals originate from the medial border of the FDL tendon, pass medial to the MTP joint, plantar to DTML, and turn dorsally to insert on lateral and middle slips of long extensor (**Fig. 4**).[1,13,15,21]

FLEXOR TENDONS

At the level of the metatarsal neck, the plantar fascia divides into a superficial and deep layer. The deep layer is thick, strong, and divides into the five processes leading to the toes. At the metatarsal head, these processes divide into two slips between

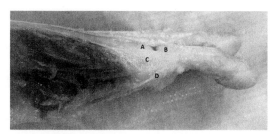

Fig. 4. Sagittal view of lesser MTP joint: A, metatarsal head; B, proximal phalanx; C, collateral ligaments; D, lumbrical tendon.

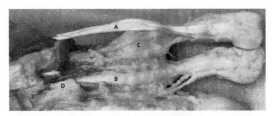

Fig. 5. Plantar view of lesser MTP joints: A, dislocated flexor tendons; B, flexor tendons in situ within tendon sheath and pulleys; C, plantar surface of plantar plate; D, plantar fascia.

which the FDL and FDB emerge.[16] After the flexor tendons emerge between these slips of plantar fascia, they pass through a fibrous tunnel and lie on the central aspect of the plantar surface of the plantar plate.[3,15] A pulley system analogous to that of the hand overlies the flexor tendons to prevent bowstringing.[23,24] The FDL and FDB tendons insert at the bases of the distal and middle phalanges, respectively. FDL and FDB flex the lesser toes to assist with gripping the ground during ambulation and push the body forward during toe-off at the end of the stance phase of the gait cycle. FDL also acts as a secondary plantarflexor of the foot at the ankle (**Fig. 5**).[16]

DEEP TRANSVERSE INTERMETATARSAL LIGAMENT

The DTML has connections on the medial and lateral sides of the plantar plate.[1] It plays a significant role in stabilizing the MTP joint and is a static restraint to dorsal subluxation of the lesser MTP joints.[25] Wang and colleagues[25] performed a sectioning study of the DTML and found that when the DTML is transected on one side of the plantar plate, resistance to dorsiflexion decreases by 17.3%. Transection of the DTML on the other side of the plantar plate results in a further decrease of 5.8%.

SUMMARY

Traditionally, the foot has been considered a tripod with most body weight distributed between the heel and the first and fifth metatarsal heads,[4] but pedobarographic studies have challenged this notion.[9–11] The plantar plate and collateral ligaments act as static stabilizers and attenuation or rupture of the static stabilizers may lead to imbalance of the MTP joint.[1,3,12,14,18–20] The flexor and extensor tendons move the toes at the MTP joints and are also dynamic stabilizers.[1,3,13,15,21–24] When treating pathology of the lesser MTP joints surgically and nonoperatively, command of the anatomy and physiology of these joints is critical.

REFERENCES

1. Nery C, Coughlin MJ, Baumfeld D, et al. Lesser metatarsal phalangeal joint arthroscopy: anatomic description and comparative dissection. Arthroscopy 2014;30(8):971–9.
2. Ridola CG, Cappello F, Marcianò V, et al. The synovial joints of the human foot. Ital J Anat Embryol 2007;112(2):61–80.
3. Nery C, Baumfeld D, Umans H, et al. MR imaging of the plantar plate: normal anatomy, turf toe, and other injuries. Magn Reson Imaging Clin N Am 2017; 25(1):127–44.
4. Cotton FJ. Foot statics and surgery. N Engl J Med 1936;214(8):353–62.

5. Arunakul M, Amendola A, Gao Y, et al. Tripod index: a new radiographic parameter assessing foot alignment. Foot Ankle Int 2013;34(10):1411–20.
6. Rodgers MM, Cavanagh PR. Pressure distribution in Morton's foot structure. Med Sci Sports Exerc 1989;21(1):23–8.
7. Weber JR, Aubin PM, Ledoux WR, et al. Second metatarsal length is positively correlated with increased pressure and medial deviation of the second toe in a robotic cadaveric simulation of gait. Foot Ankle Int 2012;33(4):312–9.
8. Chauhan D, Bhutta MA, Barrie JL. Does it matter how we measure metatarsal length? Foot Ankle Surg 2011;17(3):124–7.
9. Menz HB, Fotoohabadi MR, Munteanu SE, et al. Plantar pressures and relative lesser metatarsal lengths in older people with and without forefoot pain. J Orthop Res 2013;31(3):427–33.
10. Kanatli U, Yetkin H, Bolukbasi S. Evaluation of the transverse metatarsal arch of the foot with gait analysis. Arch Orthop Trauma Surg 2003;123(4):148–50.
11. Kaipel M, Krapf D, Wyss C. Metatarsal length does not correlate with maximal peak pressure and maximal force. Clin Orthop Relat Res 2011;469(4):1161–6.
12. Deland JT, Lee KT, Sobel M, et al. Anatomy of the plantar plate and its attachments in the lesser metatarsal phalangeal joint. Foot Ankle Int 1995;16(8):480–6.
13. Maas NM, van der Grinten M, Bramer WM, et al. Metatarsophalangeal joint stability: a systematic review on the plantar plate of the lesser toes. J Foot Ankle Res 2016;9:32.
14. Suero EM, Meyers KN, Bohne WH. Stability of the metatarsophalangeal joint of the lesser toes: a cadaveric study. J Orthop Res 2012;30(12):1995–8.
15. Johnston RB, Smith J, Daniels T. The plantar plate of the lesser toes: an anatomical study in human cadavers. Foot Ankle Int 1994;15(5):276–82.
16. Stainsby GD. Pathological anatomy and dynamic effect of the displaced plantar plate and the importance of the integrity of the plantar plate-deep transverse metatarsal ligament tie-bar. Ann R Coll Surg Engl 1997;79(1):58–68.
17. Gregg J, Marks P, Silberstein M, et al. Histologic anatomy of the lesser metatarsophalangeal joint plantar plate. Surg Radiol Anat 2007;29(2):141–7.
18. Deland JT, Sung IH. The medial crosssover toe: a cadaveric dissection. Foot Ankle Int 2000;21(5):375–8.
19. Barg A, Courville XF, Nickisch F, et al. Role of collateral ligaments in metatarsophalangeal stability: a cadaver study. Foot Ankle Int 2012;33(10):877–82.
20. Bhatia D, Myerson MS, Curtis MJ, et al. Anatomical restraints to dislocation of the second metatarsophalangeal joint and assessment of a repair technique. J Bone Joint Surg Am 1994;76(9):1371–5.
21. Sarrafian SK, Topouzian LK. Anatomy and physiology of the extensor apparatus of the toes. J Bone Joint Surg Am 1969;51(4):669–79.
22. Dalmau-Pastor M, Fargues B, Alcolea E, et al. Extensor apparatus of the lesser toes: anatomy with clinical implications: topical review. Foot Ankle Int 2014; 35(10):957–69.
23. Martin MG, Masear VR. Triggering of the lesser toes at a previously undescribed distal pulley system. Foot Ankle Int 1998;19(2):113–7.
24. Tafur M, Iwasaki K, Statum S, et al. Magnetic resonance imaging of the pulleys of the flexor tendons of the toes at 11.7 T. Skeletal Radiol 2015;44(1):87–95.
25. Wang B, Guss A, Chalayon O, et al. Deep transverse metatarsal ligament and static stability of lesser metatarsophalangeal joints: a cadaveric study. Foot Ankle Int 2015;36(5):573–8.

Conservative Management of Metatarsalgia and Lesser Toe Deformities

Andrew E. Federer, MD, David M. Tainter, MD,
Samuel B. Adams, MD, Karl M. Schweitzer Jr, MD*

KEYWORDS

- Metatarsalgia • Hammer toe • Claw toe • Mallet toe • Crossover toe • Forefoot pain

KEY POINTS

- Primary metatarsalgia is caused by abnormalities in anatomy, relationships between metatarsals, and between metatarsals and other parts of the foot that may overload the metatarsals.
- Secondary metatarsalgia is caused by conditions that affect the metatarsals directly because of trauma, indirectly through systemic conditions, or conditions that cause forefoot overload.
- Much of the current nonoperative management relies on shoewear modification, orthoses, and inserts, which work to alleviate pain by padding and protecting prominences and limiting direct pressure at these surfaces during various points in the gait cycle.
- The goals of treatment are to relieve patient symptoms and correct the cause if possible. Initial, nonsurgical options include proper footwear, orthotics, and physical therapy. In select cases, injections are considered.

INTRODUCTION

Metatarsalgia is a general term for pain of the metatarsal. Although it is often used to describe any forefoot pain, metatarsalgia more distinctly refers to plantar-based pain at the second, third, and fourth metatarsal heads. Conservative management revolves around relieving pressure and correcting deformity through various means.[1]

METATARSALGIA PATHOPHYSIOLOGY

There are several forefoot conditions that can result in metatarsal head pain, as described later in this article. There can also be a predisposition for metatarsal pain

The authors have nothing to disclose.
Foot and Ankle Division, Department of Orthopedic Surgery, Duke University Medical Center, 2301 Erwin Road, Box 3000, Durham, NC 27710, USA
* Corresponding author.
E-mail address: karl.schweitzer@duke.edu

Foot Ankle Clin N Am 23 (2018) 9–20
https://doi.org/10.1016/j.fcl.2017.09.003
foot.theclinics.com

throughout various points of the gait cycle based on intrinsic and extrinsic imbalances. Metatarsalgia can further be classified according to primary, secondary, or iatrogenic causes.

Metatarsalgia Throughout Gait Cycle

Abnormal biomechanics in the gait cycle can result in metatarsal pain and are identified in the different stages of the gait cycle. The swing phase constitutes 40% of the gait cycle, starting at toe off and ending at heel strike. During this time the lower extremity elevates to provide proper foot clearance. Normal ankle dorsiflexion, which is 20°, is needed for foot clearance, with the tibialis anterior muscle providing the greatest dorsiflexion force. The remaining extensors work to create an eversion moment to balance the inversion force imparted by the tibialis anterior muscle.[2] Patients with inadequate dorsiflexion rely on excessive recruitment of the extrinsic toe extensors to achieve maximal dorsiflexion during the swing phase. The inability to attain normal dorsiflexion can be caused by a weak tibialis anterior, Achilles tightness, or other anatomic and biomechanical abnormalities (ie, hindfoot varus, cavus foot, and anterior tibiotalar impingement).[3] This overrecruitment of lesser toe extensors can significantly contribute to metatarsophalangeal (MTP) joint pathology by moving the fat pad distally.[4]

The stance phase constitutes 60% of the gait cycle and is further subdivided into three different "rocker" phases. In the initialization of the stance phase, which accounts for 10% of the total gait cycle, the heel acts as the first rocker. Metatarsalgia in this setting occurs because of congenital deformity, cavus foot, or a tight heel cord.[5] In the subsequent stance phase stage, the ankle acts as the second rocker, which accounts for 20% of the gait cycle. During this stage the foot remains flat on the ground; however, limited ankle motion and excessively plantarflexed lesser metatarsals may produce second rocker metatarsalgia. During the third and final rocker stage of the stance phase, making up 30% of the gait cycle, only the forefoot is in contact with the ground. Here, the MTP joints are already dorsiflexed, therefore any progressive deformity is reinforced during this stage. This results in third rocker metatarsalgia and is the most common form throughout the gait cycle.

Primary Metatarsalgia

Primary metatarsalgia pertains to metatarsal pain caused by abnormalities in anatomy, relationships between metatarsals, and between metatarsals and other parts of the foot that may overload the metatarsals (**Figs. 1** and **2**).[5] The most common example of this is a long second metatarsal, although there is some controversy on this in the literature.[6–8] Other common primary causes of metatarsalgia include excessive plantar flexion of the metatarsal, which can be congenital as in the case of a cavus foot or neurologic. Insufficiency of the first ray can result in dynamic transfer of pressure to the lesser metatarsals and can be caused by progressive metatarsus primus cavus, brachymetatarasia, hypermobility of the first metatarsocuneiform joint, and flatfoot. Forefoot equinus, whether from congenital abnormality, cavus foot, or heel cord contracture, also results in compensatory hyperextension of the MTP joints and increased subsequent pressures under the metatarsal heads. Similarly, deformities of the metatarsal heads themselves may result in undue pressure at this location.

Secondary Metatarsalgia

Secondary types of metatarsalgia are caused by conditions that affect the metatarsals directly because of trauma, indirectly through systemic conditions, or conditions that cause forefoot overload (**Figs. 3–5**).

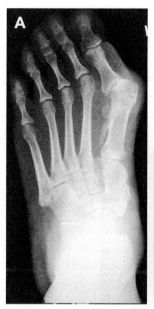
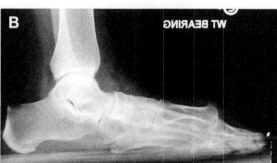

Fig. 1. Anteroposterior (*A*) and lateral (*B*) foot radiographs of a patient with pronation deformity and hallux valgus, but more notably, an insufficient first ray with hypermobility at the first tarsometatarsal joint, along with first metatarsophalangeal subluxation in both planes. This creates a long second metatarsal and transfer metatarsalgia symptoms at the lesser metatarsophalangeal joints.

Hallux rigidus is a condition of the first MTP joint that has etiology in osteoarthritis, posttraumatic, or an elevated first metatarsal. It indirectly affects the forefoot, shortens the midstance phase, and causes early heel lift off along with premature supination in the third rocker stage, resulting in transfer of pressure to the lesser metatarsal heads.

Hallux valgus also can present with metatarsalgia. Larger intermetatarsal angles may result in a long second metatarsal and higher plantar pressures. Severe hallux

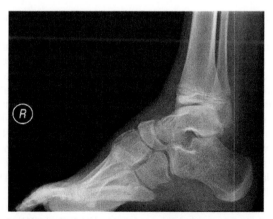

Fig. 2. Lateral foot radiograph demonstrating an adolescent with a neurologic cavovarus foot with excessive metatarsal plantarflexion, particularly at the first metatarsal, which can lead to primary metatarsalgia.

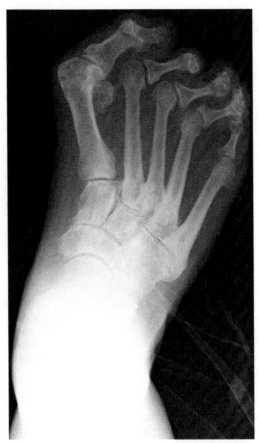

Fig. 3. Anteroposterior foot radiograph of a patient with rheumatoid arthritis demonstrating severe hallux valgus deformity with lateral subluxation of all metatarsophalangeal joints and clawing of the lesser toes, which can lead to secondary metatarsalgia.

valgus can dislocate the second toe, displacing the fat pad distally and similarly cause increased plantar pressures at the second metatarsal head.

MTP joint instability can occur from inflammatory and systemic arthropathies (eg, gout, rheumatoid arthritis), and traumatically from plantar plate rupture and postsurgical iatrogenic causes. MTP joint instability is most commonly caused by insufficiency of the plantar plate and capsule, resulting in dorsal subluxation of the joint. The second and third MTP joints are most commonly involved. A hammer toe deformity is a common concurrent condition. In addition to the dorsal instability, medial deviation is common because of lateral collateral ligament attenuation. Lateral deviation is more common with hallux valgus deformity. The "drawer test" is particularly useful to identify an unstable MTP joint. The metatarsal head is held steady by the examiner while the toe proximal phalanx is translated dorsally. Pain elicited with this maneuver is considered a positive result.

Neurologic pain is typically caused by interdigital or Morton neuroma, classically at the third webspace, and tarsal tunnel syndrome. The interdigital nerves lie between the metatarsal heads, plantar to the transverse intermetatarsal ligament. Interdigital neuromas are most common in the second and third webspaces. Patients typically

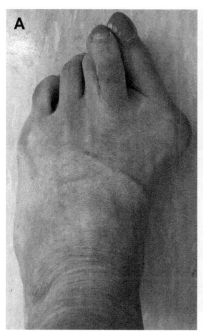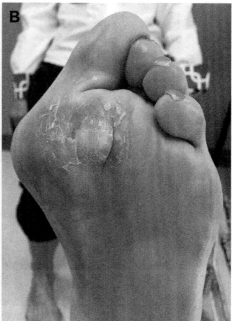

Fig. 4. Clinical photographs, including dorsal (*A*) and plantar (*B*) views, of a patient with a severe hallux valgus and lesser toe deformities, particularly a dorsally dislocated second metatarsophalangeal joint and resulting hammer toe deformity that presented with transfer metatarsalgia pain caused by overload at the plantar aspect of the second toe, evidenced by the heavy, callus formation at plantar forefoot.

complain with pain that is worse with narrower shoes. Palpating the webspace may reveal a palpable neuroma or recreate the patient's pain. Mulder click is a particularly useful maneuver where the metatarsal heads are compressed together in the examiner's hand. A positive result is a painful click. The "drawer test" should be performed to rule out a plantar plate injury.

Freiberg infraction, at its most basic level, is osteonecrosis of a metatarsal head. It most commonly involves the second metatarsal head and can have multiple etiologies. Freiberg[9] in his initial series of six patients attributed it to trauma. Since then, other causes, such as repetitive microstress, vascular compromise, diabetes mellitus, autoimmune disorders, and hypercoagulable states, have been postulated.[10] Patients typically present with localized pain over the affected metatarsals; typically the second or third metatarsals are affected. There is a significant female predisposition to this disease and the patient may report the sensation of walking on a marble or pebble, with inability to walk barefoot. Anteroposterior and oblique radiographs of the foot are most useful for appreciating the characteristic metatarsal head flattening that is pathognomonic for this condition.

Iatrogenic Metatarsalgia

Iatrogenic metatarsalgia can arise from increased forefoot pressure at the level of the lesser metatarsal heads and may be more common than previously suspected. Excessive plantar translation created from shortening metatarsal osteotomies can result in increased plantar forefoot pressure with weightbearing.[11] One of the more common

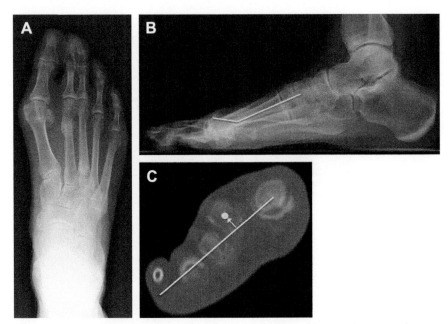

Fig. 5. Anteroposterior (*A*) and lateral (*B*) foot radiographs and coronal computed tomography cut (*C*) at the level of the metatarsophalangeal joints that demonstrates a patient who presented with discomfort and plantar callus under her third metatarsophalangeal joint after a dorsiflexion malunion of a prior second metatarsal stress fracture and existing hallux valgus deformity. This imbalance in her metatarsal cascade, primarily caused by the relative dorsal position of the second metatarsal head, as demonstrated by the *drawn lines* (*B, C*), creates transfer metatarsalgia symptoms.

causes is excessive shortening of the second metatarsal. A similar phenomenon occurs after partial metatarsal head or proximal phalangeal resections. Failed hallux valgus correction can abnormally shift plantar pressure to the lesser MTP joints (**Fig. 6**).

NONOPERATIVE MANAGEMENT OF METATARSALGIA

Although there is minimal evidence-based research to guide the optimal treatment of metatarsalgia, most patients are managed successfully in conservative fashion.

Standard nonoperative methods, such as nonsteroidal anti-inflammatory medications and activity modifications, should be part of any treatment plan, if appropriate for the specific patient. Other modes of nonsurgical treatment involve shoe modifications and toe/forefoot devices, callus shaving, corticosteroid injections (CSI), and physical therapy.

Shoewear and Orthotics

Proper footwear is essential to the treatment of metatarsalgia, especially if the current footwear contributes to the symptomatology. Shoes with an elevated heel may place increased load on the metatarsal heads. Proper footwear for treating metatarsalgia includes shoes with a wide toe box, proper length, cushioned sole, and a lowered heel.[5] Patients with hallux valgus and lesser toes deformities and webspace neuromas stand

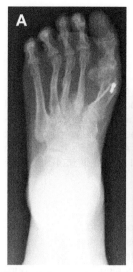
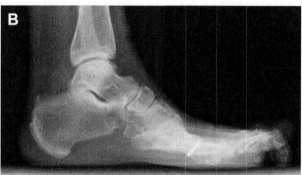

Fig. 6. Anteroposterior (*A*) and lateral (*B*) foot radiographs of a patient who presented with persisting pain under the lesser metatarsophalangeal joints that is likely attributable to malunion of prior bunion repair with significant shortening and angulation of the first metatarsal, along with further disruption of the metatarsal cascade from a shortened third metatarsal fracture malunion.

to benefit from these modifications. Athletic running shoes often have a slight rocker bottom sole, and this can provide good pain relief.[12]

Shoewear modifications and orthoses work to alleviate areas of pressure on bony prominences of the foot, producing pain relief. Orthotics with a metatarsal pad have been shown to reduce plantar pressures over the metatarsal heads. A metatarsal pad placed 6.5 mm proximal to the second metatarsal head was shown to reduce peak pressures by 33%.[13] In addition, thicker insoles were shown to provide improved pressure relief. A 12.5-mm insole further reduced peak metatarsal head pressures by 23% as compared with a 2.5-mm insole. Insoles should be worn in a shoe with proper depth to accommodate the added height. Athletes with metatarsalgia may prefer increased forefoot cushioning compared with a metatarsal pad while running. Peak pressures under the metatarsal heads were reduced by 11% during running with forefoot-cushioned orthotics as compared with standard insoles or those with a metatarsal pad.[14]

Rocker soles can also help alleviate pain from metatarsalgia. Although the term rocker sole may conjure undesirable images in a patient's mind, most modern, well-cushioned running shoes use a rocker sole concept.[12] Patients with more severe deformity or issues may require a more elaborate rocker sole. Brown and colleagues[15] showed that toe-only rockers reduced pressure under the second metatarsal head by more than 54% and by 25% under the third and fourth metatarsals. Negative heel rockers and double rockers also reduce pressure under the metatarsal heads, but by a lesser degree.

Callus Shaving

Chronic plantar keratosis is common among patients with metatarsal head pain. Conservative symptom management is performed with a callus file, pumice stones, scalpel, or callus blade. This is a simple and effective means of managing this painful condition, although treatment also needs to focus on the primary cause for metatarsalgia.

Physical Therapy

Heel cord and triceps surae tightness in the form of equinus contracture is a contributing cause of metatarsalgia. Physical therapy programs focus on a variety of heel cord and calf stretches, along with other modalities, with the aim to decrease forefoot pressure. In a study evaluating the effect of a 6-week stretching course, it was found that ankle dorsiflexion increased, passive Achilles tendon length increased, and passive resistive properties through the full range of motion of the ankle decreased.[16]

Injections

CSI can help deliver effective analgesia to the site of forefoot pain, and serve as a diagnostic and therapeutic intervention. Thomson and colleagues[17] demonstrated symptom improvement for up to 3 months in patients with interdigital neuromas who received CSIs in a patient-blinded randomized trial. Patients also need to be counseled on the risks of injection therapy. In patients with MTP joint synovitis, repeated CSIs into the joint can result in capsular and ligamentous attrition and resulting joint instability. Fat pad atrophy has been reported in patients undergoing repeated injections into plantar tissues, which could exacerbate pain at the metatarsal heads. Because of these risks, CSIs should be used in moderation and with appropriate counseling.

Sclerosing ethanol injections have been attempted to chemically ablate Morton neuromas. Hughes and colleagues[18] originally described ethanol injections into the affected webspace of 101 patients with 94% of patients experiencing relief of their symptoms and 84% experiencing complete resolution. However, the average follow-up in the study was only 10.5 months. More recently, Gurdezi and coworkers[19] reported 5-year follow-up data for alcohol injections. Results at 5 years were moderate at best, with only 29% of patients reporting symptom relief. In that study, 36% of patients went on to surgical excision at an average of 2 years postinjection. Animal models of Morton neuromas reveal that sclerosing alcohol injections were safe to administer and histologic analysis revealed no evidence of neural necrosis, apoptosis, or inflammatory response related to the injections.[20]

In a randomized-controlled trial, ultrasound guidance used for webspace injections conferred no benefit over nonguided injections.[21] Hembree and colleagues[22] showed that fellowship-trained orthopedic surgeons injected interdigital neuromas with 100% accuracy using only anatomic landmarks. Ultrasound guidance is generally not required by experienced surgeons but may be useful for diagnosis or in the hands of the less experienced providers.

Protected Weight Bearing

Certain causes of metatarsalgia, such as Freiberg infraction, should be treated conservatively with a period of immobilization and limited weight bearing. In Freiberg infraction, limited weight bearing and immobilization may not only relieve painful symptoms but may also limit destruction to the MTP joint. Depending on patient compliance, this is done with a cast, boot, or a stiff-soled shoe. Morandi and colleagues[23] described a form of immobilization and skeletal traction with a short leg cast that decreased pain symptoms in patients. Unlike avascular necrosis of the femoral head, the role of bisphosponates in Freiberg infraction has not been studied, and thus cannot be recommended.[10]

PATHOPHYSIOLOGY OF OTHER LESSER TOE ABNORMALITIES
Mallet Toes

A mallet toe is a deformity characterized by flexion of the distal interphalangeal (DIP) joint and neutral position of the proximal interphalangeal (PIP) and MTP joints. Often caused by pressure inside a shoe, the flexor digitorum longus tendon may eventually contract resulting in fixed deformity. A similar presentation may occur from extensor digitorum longus laceration or rupture at the level of the DIP joint.

Hammer Toes

Hammer toes are characterized by a flexed PIP joint, typically with extension of the DIP joint and a neutral or more rarely a hyperextended MTP joint. Although hammer toes may involve either DIP joint flexion or MTP joint extension in conjunction with PIP joint flexion deformity, the presence of all three joint deformities in the same toe is referred to as a claw toe. A hammer toe deformity must be evaluated carefully because it frequently occurs in conjunction with other conditions, such as MTP joint instability. Plain film radiographs are helpful in detecting associated conditions, such as MTP joint subluxation, dislocation, and long metatarsals.

Claw Toes

A claw toe deformity is distinguished by flexion at the PIP and DIP joints with concomitant extension at the MTP joint. In comparison with its oft confused relative, the hammer toe, a claw toe deformity is less common but more severe. The basis of this deformity is an overpowering of the intrinsic forces by the extrinsic forces. Namely, the extensor digitorum longus tendon pulls on the extensor sling causing MTP joint hyperextension. This, in conjunction with rotation of the intrinsic muscles, creates a deforming force further inducing MTP joint hyperextension, which can also occur through loss of plantar MTP joint stability.[24] With the MTP joint in extension and intrinsic muscles weakened, the flexor digitorum brevis and flexor digitorum longus tendons are tensioned, causing flexion at the PIP and DIP joints. A profound imbalance of intrinsic and extrinsic muscles is a primary cause of claw toe deformities, therefore in certain patients, a neurologic evaluation is warranted.

CONSERVATIVE MANAGEMENT OF MALLET, HAMMER, AND CLAW TOES

Mallet toes result in impaction of the distal phalanx and nail into the ground. Conservative management for mallet toes involves relieving pressure at the distal tip of the phalanx, through the use of cushioned foam, gel sleeves, and/or toe crest devices, which are helpful because they elevate the toe, keeping the toe tip offloaded. Callus trimming, placement of a felt pad, and using shoes with a wide toe box and deepened heel can also reduce pressure and alleviate symptoms.

The conservative treatment of hammer and claw toes is similar, with consideration on whether these are flexible or rigid deformities and focus on alleviating the pressure on the dorsum of the PIP joint, and also under the MTP joint. Shoe modification is the first line of treatment, which focuses on a widened and taller toe box and shoes with increased depth to allow free movement of the PIP joint dorsally. A toe crest also can be used. Doughnut cutouts can help redistribute plantar joint pressure, whereas foam or gel toe sleeves cushion the flexed PIP joint against the inside of the shoe, which is useful in a more rigid deformity. A Budin splint is a flat pad with an elastic strap dorsally that is designed to reduce a flexible interphalangeal joint deformity, allowing the toe to rest in a more neutral position (**Fig. 7**). Taping of the proximal phalanx in a figure-of-eight pattern can help prevent MTP subluxation and reduce flexible deformity.

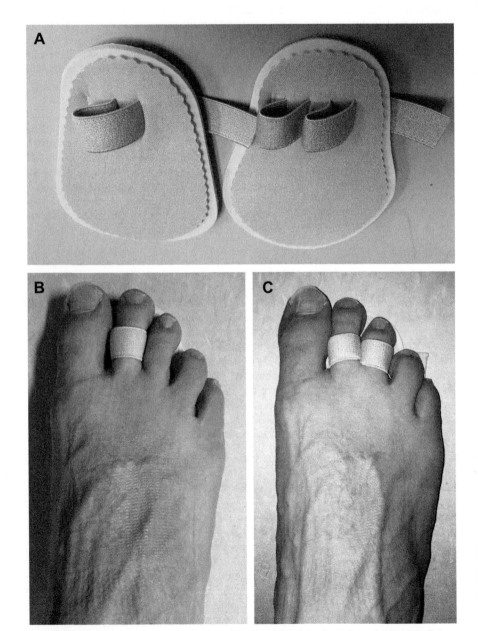

Fig. 7. (A) Photograph of a single (*left*) and double (*right*) Budin splint, along with demonstration of the use of single (*B*) and double (*C*) Budin splints for flexible hammer toe deformities to help hold the affected toes in relative straightened positions.

SUMMARY

The causes of metatarsalgia and lesser toe deformities are many and initial management should consist of nonoperative measures. Nonoperative management consists of proper footwear. Orthoses or physical therapy may be useful for many patients. Injections and protected weight bearing should be undertaken only in select cases and after discussion of risks and benefits with the patient. An in-depth understanding of the various etiologies of metatarsalgia and lesser toe deformities is essential to successful treatment.

REFERENCES

1. Shirzad K, Kiesau CD, DeOrio JK, et al. Lesser toe deformities. J Am Acad Orthop Surg 2011;19(8):505–14.
2. Gopfert B, Valderrabano V, Hintermann B, et al. Measurement of the isometric dorsiflexion and plantar flexion force in the ankle joint. Biomed Tech (Berl) 2005;50(9):282–6 [in German].
3. Aronow MS, Diaz-Doran V, Sullivan RJ, et al. The effect of triceps surae contracture force on plantar foot pressure distribution. Foot Ankle Int 2006;27(1):43–52.
4. Espinosa N, Maceira E, Myerson MS. Current concept review: metatarsalgia. Foot Ankle Int 2008;29(8):871–9.
5. Espinosa N, Brodsky JW, Maceira E. Metatarsalgia. J Am Acad Orthop Surg 2010;18(8):474–85.
6. Maestro M, Besse JL, Ragusa M, et al. Forefoot morphotype study and planning method for forefoot osteotomy. Foot Ankle Clin 2003;8(4):695–710.
7. Menz HB, Fotoohabadi MR, Munteanu SE, et al. Plantar pressures and relative lesser metatarsal lengths in older people with and without forefoot pain. J Orthop Res 2013;31(3):427–33.
8. Kaipel M, Krapf D, Wyss C. Metatarsal length does not correlate with maximal peak pressure and maximal force. Clin Orthop Relat Res 2011;469(4):1161–6.
9. Freiberg AH. Infraction of the second metatarsal bone, a typical injury. Surg Gynecol Obstet 1914;(19):191–6.
10. Cerrato RA. Freiberg's disease. Foot Ankle Clin 2011;16(4):647–58.
11. Acevedo JI. Fixation of metatarsal osteotomies in the treatment of hallux valgus. Foot Ankle Clin 2000;5(3):451–68.
12. Janisse DJ, Janisse E. Shoe modification and the use of orthoses in the treatment of foot and ankle pathology. J Am Acad Orthop Surg 2008;16(3):152–8.
13. Chen WM, Lee SJ, Lee PV. Plantar pressure relief under the metatarsal heads: therapeutic insole design using three-dimensional finite element model of the foot. J Biomech 2015;48(4):659–65.
14. Hahni M, Hirschmuller A, Baur H. The effect of foot orthoses with forefoot cushioning or metatarsal pad on forefoot peak plantar pressure in running. J Foot Ankle Res 2016;9:44.
15. Brown D, Wertsch JJ, Harris GF, et al. Effect of rocker soles on plantar pressures. Arch Phys Med Rehabil 2004;85(1):81–6.
16. Gajdosik RL, Allred JD, Gabbert HL, et al. A stretching program increases the dynamic passive length and passive resistive properties of the calf muscle-tendon unit of unconditioned younger women. Eur J Appl Physiol 2007;99(4):449–54.
17. Thomson CE, Beggs I, Martin DJ, et al. Methylprednisolone injections for the treatment of Morton neuroma: a patient-blinded randomized trial. J Bone Joint Surg Am 2013;95(9):790–8, s791.

18. Hughes RJ, Ali K, Jones H, et al. Treatment of Morton's neuroma with alcohol injection under sonographic guidance: follow-up of 101 cases. Am J Roentgenol 2007;188(6):1535–9.
19. Gurdezi S, White T, Ramesh P. Alcohol injection for Morton's neuroma: a five-year follow-up. Foot Ankle Int 2013;34(8):1064–7.
20. Mazoch MJ, Cheema GA, Suva LJ, et al. Effects of alcohol injection in rat sciatic nerve as a model for Morton's neuroma treatment. Foot Ankle Int 2014;35(11): 1187–91.
21. Mahadevan D, Attwal M, Bhatt R, et al. Corticosteroid injection for Morton's neuroma with or without ultrasound guidance: a randomised controlled trial. Bone Joint J 2016;98-b(4):498–503.
22. Hembree WC, Groth AT, Schon LC, et al. Computed tomography analysis of third webspace injections for interdigital neuroma. Foot Ankle Int 2013;34(4):575–8.
23. Morandi A, Prina A, Verdoni F. The treatment of Kohler's second syndrome by continuous skeletal traction. Ital J Orthop Traumatol 1990;16(3):363–8.
24. Myerson MS, Shereff MJ. The pathological anatomy of claw and hammer toes. J Bone Joint Surg Am 1989;71(1):45–9.

Treatment of Metatarsalgia with Distal Osteotomies

David Redfern, FRCS (Tr&Orth)

KEYWORDS

- Metatarsalgia • Distal osteotomies • Percutaneous osteotomies • Forefoot

KEY POINTS

- Many different distal metatarsal osteotomies have been described in the surgical treatment of metatarsalgia.
- The surgeon should use such osteotomies judiciously, and indeed, in this author's experience, they are infrequently required and are certainly not a first port of call.
- In cases where nonoperative treatments have failed, a thorough understanding of the causes of metatarsalgia and a detailed clinical assessment of the patient are essential if good surgical outcomes are to be achieved.
- If using distal metatarsal osteotomies as part of the surgical plan, then this author favors extra-articular percutaneous osteotomies to minimize postoperative stiffness.

INTRODUCTION

Metatarsalgia is a symptom and not a diagnosis. It simply describes pain on the plantar aspect of the forefoot in the metatarsal head region (ie, the "ball of the foot"). The skill therefore lies in diagnosis of the cause or causes of this pain. Not until the cause or causes have been identified can the surgeon then consider appropriate treatment. It may sound obvious but the causes of metatarsalgia are numerous and can be interrelated. Not until a surgeon is skilled in the assessment of metatarsalgia can they hope to be successful in its treatment.

Although the term metatarsalgia itself does not distinguish between first and lesser metatarsal head region pain, the scope of this article is limited to the treatment of this symptom in the lesser rays.

As a rule, distal metatarsal osteotomies should be used sparingly in the treatment of metatarsalgia. The persistence of metatarsalgia despite nonoperative treatment does not automatically imply the need to use distal metatarsal osteotomies. In general, the surgeon should aim to correct the underlying cause of the metatarsalgia.

The author has nothing to disclose.
London Foot and Ankle Centre, Hospital St John & St Elizabeth, 60 Grove End Road, London, NW8 9NH, UK
E-mail address: davidjredfern@me.com

Foot Ankle Clin N Am 23 (2018) 21–33
https://doi.org/10.1016/j.fcl.2017.09.004
1083-7515/18/© 2017 Elsevier Inc. All rights reserved.

For example, the patient presenting with metatarsalgia in the presence of hallux valgus rarely requires distal metatarsal osteotomies unless there is associated lesser metatarsophalangeal joint (MTPJ) subluxation/dislocation. Adequate triplanar correction of the hallux valgus deformity will restore the windlass mechanism and function of the first ray. Restoration of the Windlass mechanism will in turn will almost always sufficiently reduce lesser ray loading such that lesser metatarsal surgery is not required. This is not an absolute rule but one that generally holds true in this author's practice.

CAUSES OF METATARSALGIA

- Biomechanical
  - Trauma
  - Iatrogenic
  - Congenital
- Biological
  - Metabolic
  - Infection
  - Neoplastic

MEDIATORS OF METATARSALGIA

- *Lesser MTPJs* (synovitis, degenerative change, plantar plate abnormality)
- *Metatarsal heads* (stress response, fracture, avascular necrosis)
- *Sesamoids* (stress response, fracture, degenerative change, avascular necrosis)
- *Interdigital neuromas* (usually secondary to biomechanical abnormality)
- *Other plantar soft tissue* (skin corns/callosities/scars, bursitis, flexor tenosynovitis, plantar fibroma)

BIOMECHANICAL CAUSES OF METATARSALGIA

- Secondary forefoot overload
  - Hindfoot and/or ankle deformity
  - Gastroc soleus contracture
- First ray abnormality
  - Hallux valgus
  - Hallux rigidus
  - Iatrogenic disturbance
- Metatarsal cascade abnormality
  - Sagittal plane deformity
  - Coronal plane deformity
  - Iatrogenic disturbance
- Lesser toe deformity
  - Usually itself secondary to proximal abnormality (see earlier discussion)

CLINICAL EVALUATION

As has already been emphasized, a thorough history and detailed examination (standing and lying) including the knee, working distally to the toes and including footwear, are vital in evaluating the cause or causes of metatarsalgia. This has been emphasized and detailed by other investigators.[1–3] Radiographic examination with weight-bearing anteroposterior and lateral views of the foot is obligatory, and a skyline metatarsal view can also be helpful in assessing metatarsal sagittal inclination. Ultrasound, MRI, and computed tomography (CT) scan (including weight-bearing CT) investigations may also be helpful in more complex cases. Pedobarography is not part of this author's routine initial assessment but can also be helpful in complex cases and for documentation in the revision situation, supporting clinical decision making.

During gait, functioning of the foot has been described as a 3-rocker system,[4] and it can be helpful to consider the causes of metatarsalgia according to these 3 rocker phases of the gait cycle.[1]

First Rocker (Heel Strike Progressing to Foot Flat on Floor)

Abnormalities such as flexion deformities of the knee and complex hindfoot deformity can cause metatarsalgia; in these cases, distal metatarsal osteotomies will not be sufficient and the underlying deformity must be addressed, for example, correction of knee flexion deformity, cavovarus deformity correction, and Achilles tendon contracture correction.

Second Rocker (Progression of the Body over the Foot with Progressive Dorsiflexion of the Ankle)

Abnormalities responsible for reduced ankle dorsiflexion or plantar-flexed metatarsals can cause metatarsalgia in the second rocker phase, and again, surgery should be directed at correction of these abnormalities, for example, correction of gastroc soleus contracture, removal of anterior ankle osteophytes, or elevation of plantar flexed metatarsals with proximal metatarsal osteotomies.

Third Rocker (The Foot Pivots over the Metatarsal Heads)

Plantar callosities tend to be more diffuse in this situation and often caused by abnormalities such as subluxed or dislocated MTPJs, lesser toe deformities, and first ray insufficiency/abnormality (eg, hallux valgus and hallux rigidus). This is the situation in which distal metatarsal osteotomies may be indicated, although this author would still generally favor avoiding them if possible. In other words, the focus should be correction of the causative abnormality, such as hallux valgus deformity, and only to use distal metatarsal osteotomies where there is absolute requirement, such as in subluxed or dislocated MTPJs or obvious severe disparity of metatarsal length/inclination. Otherwise, a comprehensive triplanar correction of the first ray abnormality is generally sufficient and will avoid the need for lesser metatarsal surgery.

It is important to remember that there may well be several factors contributing to the patient's symptoms involving more than one rocker phase, and if the patient has unilateral symptoms, then comparison with the asymptomatic limb is particularly helpful in assessing the key problem areas that must be addressed.

TYPES OF DISTAL METATARSAL OSTEOTOMY TECHNIQUES

Whichever technique a surgeon selects, the aim is to reduce the prominence and hence loading of one or more metatarsal heads. Depending on the technique used, this can be achieved by elevation, dorsiflexion, or shortening of the metatarsal (or a combination of these).

One difficulty the surgeon faces is in knowing how much displacement is sufficient to correct the biomechanical problem without transferring too much load to an adjacent metatarsal head. Another problem that follows from this is then to decide how many osteotomies to undertake and of which metatarsals.

There is a fine line between sufficient and excessive displacement, and there is no formula that can reliably predict the correct elevation/shortening required. This is more appreciable when one considers the complex elements of biomechanics that contribute to metatarsalgia in the first place (eg, gastrocnemius tension, restriction of ankle motion, overall foot architecture, footwear demands of the patient).

The surgeon needs to decide where the abnormalities lie and can then consider whether one or more distal metatarsal osteotomies are appropriate and whether further surgery such as gastrocnemius lengthening is required.

Many different operations have been reported,[1,5] and a short review of the different varieties follows here. Unfortunately, there are no high level comparative data in the literature to allow valid conclusions as to the optimum technique. However, it is vital that surgeons undertaking lesser ray osteotomies are experienced in the treatment of forefoot abnormality and the behavior, limitations, and potential pitfalls of their preferred osteotomy technique. There follows here a brief review of different osteotomy techniques.

Open Techniques

Weil osteotomy

A shortening osteotomy is shown in **Fig. 1** (distal oblique intra-articular metaphyseal metatarsal osteotomy).

Weil first described this in 1985 for the treatment of central metatarsalgia, and Barouk[6] subsequently introduced the technique to France in 1992. It has become the most popular technique of distal metatarsal osteotomy in Europe and North America.

The technique is well described elsewhere[1] and is not be described again here. Numerous modifications have been described but without evidence that they influence outcome.[1,7] In its original form, the Weil is a shortening osteotomy, but many prefer to remove a slither of bone from the osteotomy at the same time in order to introduce some elevation in addition to shortening.[1] The main reason for introducing this modification was due to concern that it is difficult to achieve an osteotomy parallel with the floor and more likely that the surgeon will create a slope in the osteotomy that will lead to plantarization of the head as it is displaces proximally. Thus, the reason for removing the slither of bone from the osteotomy is to compensate for this tendency to plantarize during shortening rather than to elevate the head as such. Evidence is lacking that this modification influences outcome.[7]

The osteotomy is usually fixed with a twist-off–type screw, versions of which are made by various orthopedic companies. How much shortening is of course the important question?

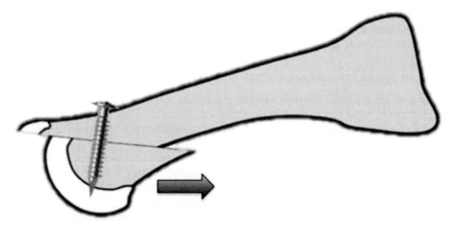

Fig. 1. Weil osteotomy.

Much emphasis has been placed on the "harmonious" foot described by Maestro and colleagues[8] in 2003 as a method of predicting adequate shortening. However, this model fails to adequately consider the sagittal plane (ie, metatarsal inclination) or any more proximal abnormality and is not predictive of clinical failures.[9] Khurna and colleagues[10] demonstrated that persistent postoperative metatarsalgia after the Weil osteotomy was associated with metatarsal plantar prominence on a metatarsal skyline radiograph.

Although good to excellent results have been reported in 70% to 100% of patients treated with conventional Weil osteotomy,[11–15] complications of MTPJ stiffness and floating-toe deformity are very common.[15,16] Other reported complications include transfer metatarsalgia, wound healing problems, and complex regional pain syndrome.[17]

Distal metatarsal "V" osteotomy

A dorsiflexion elevating osteotomy is shown in **Fig. 2** (an extra-articular metaphyseal-diaphyseal junction dorsal closing wedge osteotomy).

Meisenbach[18] and then later Thomas[19] advocated using a closing-wedge osteotomy (3 cm proximal to the MPTJ). Thomas published the results of 73 osteotomies in 39 rheumatoid feet using this technique and reported pain relief in 90%. Wolf[20] described a V-shaped closing wedge osteotomy 4 to 6 cm proximal to the metatarsal head.

Leventen and Pearson described a V-shaped osteotomy (apex plantar) at the metaphyseal-diaphyseal junction as a modification of technique described by Wolf, which was undertaken in the distal diaphysis.[20–23] In an effort to avoid transfer lesions,

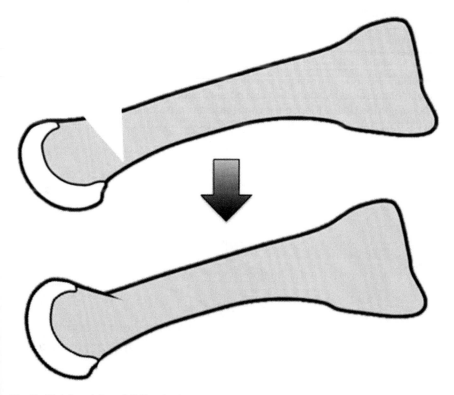

Fig. 2. Distal metatarsal "V" osteotomy.

they also described an algorithm to determine which metatarsals to osteotomize depending on the site of the callous. The osteotomy involved making a V-shaped trough in the metatarsal neck with a rongeur. This was then closed in a dorsal direction with manual pressure without fixation. They reported their results in 21 feet with this technique. Nearly 25% still had residual metatarsalgia symptoms, although 18/21 reported complete or partial satisfaction with their result.

This author has no experience with this technique; also, it will not allow for correction of metatarsal length.

Distal chevron osteotomy

A predominantly dorsally translating elevating osteotomy is shown in **Fig. 3** (an extra-articular metaphyseal-diaphyseal junction dorsal translation osteotomy).

Kitaoka and Patzer[22] described a vertical plane distal chevron osteotomy (apex distal). The apex of the chevron was created using a drill at the metadiaphyseal junction of the metatarsal, and the chevron limbs were created with a microsagittal saw directed proximally at 45°. The distal fragment was displaced dorsally approximately 2 to 3 mm and manually impacted. The author used temporary Kirschner wire fixation to control the osteotomy position (wire removed at 3 weeks after surgery).

Kitaoka and Patzer published a retrospective review of a small group of 19 patients (21 feet) who had undergone 24 osteotomies with a mean follow-up of 4 years (2–7). Fifteen patients had no pain; 2 had mild pain, and 2 had moderate pain. Two patients required further surgery with moderate or severe pain. Five of the 19 feet reported no footwear limitation, but 14 feet could not tolerate fashionable shoes, and 3 of these required orthotics. No patient required a custom-made shoe, but 4 feet still had a painful plantar callosity. The overall clinical results were classified as good in 16 feet, fair in 2, and poor in 3, because of painful plantar callosities.

Other open osteotomies

Many other different osteotomies have been described. Helal[24] and subsequently Helal and Greiss[25] described an oblique osteotomy of the central 3 metatarsals for the treatment of metatarsalgia by shortening and dorsally angulating the bone. This osteotomy was popular in the United Kingdom for several years, but studies showed that this technique did not provide for a reliable outcome. Winson[26] reported disappointing results in

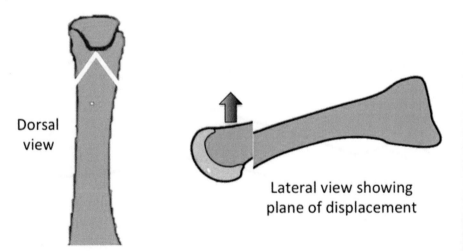

Dorsal view

Lateral view showing plane of displacement

Fig. 3. Distal chevron osteotomy.

66/124 feet reviewed at a mean of 3 years after surgery. In another study, Pedowitz[27] reported a 25% incidence of transfer lesions or residual callosities in a study group of 49 patients at a mean of 16 months after surgery. This technique is not recommended because of the large (unlimited) displacements that can occur.

Percutaneous Techniques

Distal metatarsal metaphyseal osteotomies

An elevating and shortening osteotomy is shown in **Fig. 4** (an extra-articular distal metatarsal metaphyseal oblique osteotomy).

The term distal metatarsal metaphyseal osteotomies (DMMO) is descriptive of the site of the osteotomy, and this is important in dictating its mechanical behavior. It is an extra-articular metaphyseal osteotomy. The DMMO has become popular in Europe as an alternative surgical technique to the traditional Weil osteotomy with its inherent problems of postoperative MTPJ stiffness and floating toe. There are also the perceived potential advantages of a "dynamic" correction offered by the DMMO. The term "dynamic" is used to describe the freedom of the osteotomy to move in 2 planes, allowing both elevation and shortening as dictated by the soft tissues and weight-bearing and influenced by the more proximal biomechanical elements discussed earlier.

Surgical technique The surgical technique is described in detail by this author in a previous publication in this journal.[28] The osteotomy is made via a small portal on the dorsal aspect of the foot adjacent to the MTPJ of the metatarsal to be addressed. No tourniquet is required, and any bleeding is useful for cooling the burr during the surgery. The burr (2 × 12-mm Shannon burr; Wright Medical USA) is introduced via the dorsal portal and positioned to the right-hand side of the metatarsal neck (left side if the surgeon is left-handed) at the diaphyseal-metaphyseal junction. The positioning of the burr is very important and can be confirmed on image intensifier initially, although with experience, this will not be necessary. The burr is angled at 45° to the longitudinal axis of the metatarsal, and the cut is created in a sweeping action involving a supination of the surgeon's wrist so that the cut proceeds from the right-hand side of the metatarsal metaphyseal flare, through to exit on the dorsal surface of the metaphysis (**Fig. 5**). The osteotomy is extracapsular. No fixation is required.

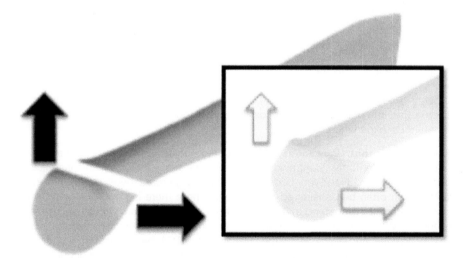

Fig. 4. DMMO.

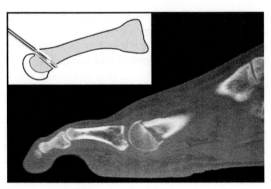

Fig. 5. Position and plane of DMMO.

The osteotomy is *only* complete when the metatarsal head is mobile in the sagittal plane *and* also telescopes in a proximal-distal plane. If both these planes of motion are not present, then there will some intact bone/periosteum limiting motion and this must be cut/freed. The position of the osteotomy and the plane in which it is made can be significantly altered if the surgeon does not adhere to the recommended technique. Relatively small changes in the position of the osteotomy and its plane can have large effects on its behavior. Cadaveric training is mandatory in this author's opinion.

When performing DMMOs, it should generally be considered obligatory to perform the osteotomies to the second, third, and fourth metatarsals in order to avoid a transfer lesion developing under the third or fourth metatarsal heads. A DMMO of the fifth should also be added in the presence of a relatively small length difference between fourth and fifth metatarsals to avoid symptoms in the fifth toe, where it will not sit comfortably against the fourth toe. Isolated DMMOs of a single metatarsal should generally be avoided but can be undertaken in specific circumstances when very experienced with this technique.

Postoperative management The patient is allowed (and encouraged) to full weight-bear immediately after surgery in a protective flat, stiff-soled postoperative shoe with crutches for support. Generally, patients report very little pain, but that which is present is usually localized to the dorsum of the forefoot. Strict elevation is required for the first 2 weeks (50 minutes of each and every hour of the day), and the patient is reviewed at 2 weeks postoperatively. At this stage, this author recommends switching the patient into a short removable pneumatic boot for a further 6 weeks (full weight-bearing). The short removable pneumatic boot provides better immobilization of the osteotomies and allows more rapid union, in this author's experience.

Indications and contraindications For this, osteotomy is broadly the same as those for the Weil osteotomy. Contraindications include active infection and insufficient vascular perfusion. However, because of the tiny percutaneous portal incisions, DMMOs can often be considered in situations where there is poor local soft tissue or previous incisions/scarring that might otherwise be of concern with larger open incisions (eg, Weil). Redfern and Vernois[28] advise against DMMO in the presence of significant arthritis and stiffness in the associated MTPJ because of the observed increased risk of nonunion in this situation (motion then predominantly occurs at the osteotomy site rather than the MTPJ).

Results Comparative studies relating to this technique versus open techniques remain sparse in the literature. Those studies that are available suggest at least equivalent results when compared with those of Weil osteotomies in the treatment of metatarsalgia.[29–31] In the opinion of this author, the lack of postoperative stiffness is the main attraction with DMMOs,[31] but the tradeoff can be more prolonged swelling in some patients and higher incidence of symptomatic delayed union, although symptoms from this are usually low level. The risk of prolonged swelling and delayed union can be reduced by placing the patient in a short pneumatic boot (full weight-bearing) from postoperative weeks 2 to 8. Symptomatic nonunion is rare (<1% in the experience of this author).

Complications The list of potential complications is the same as for an open osteotomy, including infection (<0.5%), soft tissue complications, delayed/nonunion, and malunion. Symptomatic nonunion is rare (approximately 1:500–1:1000).[32] However, delayed union is in the region of 5% and usually affects the second (or third less commonly) metatarsal osteotomies.[32]

With Weil's osteotomies, because of the rigid internal fixation, there is rarely malunion. However, with no internal fixation, DMMOs can displace during the healing period. This is likely to be due to the force exerted by the extensor digitorum brevis and can result in lateralization of the second and third metatarsal heads and almost always some medialization of the M5 head (advantageous in treating bunionette deformity with this technique). The displacement is not usually significant and rarely compromises the clinical result, but care should be taken when combining DMMOs with hallux valgus correction because the tendency for second and third metatarsal head lateralization during the postoperative period is increased.

Distal incomplete metatarsal metaphyseal oblique osteotomy
An elevating osteotomy is shown in **Fig. 6** (an extra-articular distal incomplete metatarsal metaphyseal oblique osteotomy).

The technique for this osteotomy is exactly the same as for the DMMO (described earlier) except that a slim bone bridge is left behind at the proximal

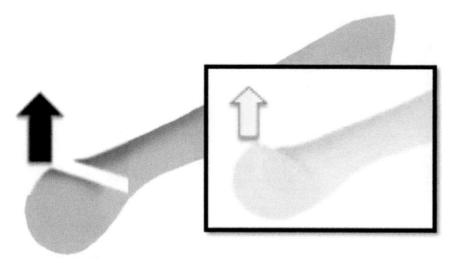

Fig. 6. Distal incomplete metatarsal metaphyseal osteotomy.

plantar extent of the osteotomy. This renders the osteotomy mobile in only one plane, allowing only sagittal plane motion (dorsiflexion). Because the burr is 2 mm in diameter, an elevation (dorsiflexion) of the metatarsal head is created as the osteotomy is closed manually. If further displacement is required, then the burr is run through the osteotomy in the same path again while manually holding the osteotomy closed.

This osteotomy can be useful where metatarsal head elevation is required without shortening.[28] There is very little postoperative swelling or pain, and a return to normal footwear is usually possible from 2 weeks after surgery.

CLINICAL EXAMPLES EMPLOYING PERCUTANEOUS TECHNIQUES
Example 1

Example 1 is a 68-year-old woman who presented with metatarsalgia accompanied by severe hallux valgus and "splay foot" (**Fig. 7**). The first MTPJ was fused to address the severe hallux valgus. This was then combined with percutaneous soft tissue release of the second and third MTPJs (extensor tenotomies, dorsal capsular release, intra-articular release of collateral ligaments), percutaneous proximal phalanx osteotomies of the second and third toes, and percutaneous DMMOs of M2-5. Note the direction of displacement of the DMMO's: in addition to shortening occurring, M2 has drifted slightly laterally, M3 is neutral, and M4 and M5 have displaced medially due to the axis of the extensor and flexor tendons, which helped to narrow the forefoot.

Example 2

Example 2 is a 55-year-old man who presented with metatarsalgia and painful hammered second toe, which had dorsally dislocated at the second MTPJ (**Fig. 8**). Note the previous stress fracture of the third metatarsal. This patient was treated with DMMOs of metatarsals 2 and 4 (not the third due to the previous stress fracture,

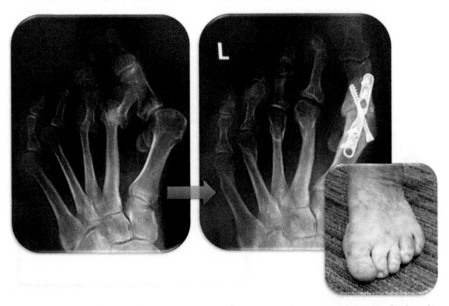

Fig. 7. Case example 1 with preoperative and postoperative anteroposterior (AP) radiographs and clinical photograph.

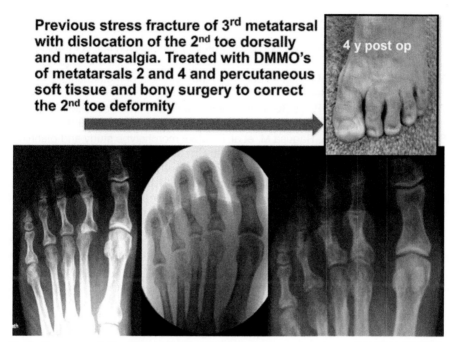

Previous stress fracture of 3rd metatarsal with dislocation of the 2nd toe dorsally and metatarsalgia. Treated with DMMO's of metatarsals 2 and 4 and percutaneous soft tissue and bony surgery to correct the 2nd toe deformity

4 y post op

Fig. 8. Case example 2 with preoperative, intraoperative, and postoperative AP radiographs and clinical photograph.

which had already elevated this) and percutaneous soft tissue and bony surgery to correct the second toe deformity. Four years later, the second toe remained reduced and the patient remained pain free.

SUMMARY

Many different distal metatarsal osteotomies have been described in the surgical treatment of metatarsalgia. The surgeon should use such osteotomies judiciously, and indeed, in this author's experience, they are infrequently required and are certainly not a first port of call. In cases where nonoperative treatments have failed, a thorough understanding of the causes of metatarsalgia and a detailed clinical assessment of the patient are essential if good surgical outcomes are to be achieved. If using distal metatarsal osteotomies as part of the surgical plan, then this author favors extra-articular percutaneous osteotomies to minimize postoperative stiffness. Proximal contributory abnormality must be recognized and adequately addressed as well as local forefoot abnormality. The surgeon should not underestimate the power of the first ray abnormality correction in treating concurrent metatarsalgia, which can often obviate lesser metatarsal surgery.

REFERENCES

1. Schuh R, Trnka HJ. Metatarsalgia: distal metatarsal osteotomies. Foot Ankle Clin N Am 2011;16:583–95.
2. Barouk P. Recurrent metatarsalgia. Foot Ankle Clin N Am 2014;19:407–24.
3. Hamilton KD, Anderson JG, Bohay DR. Current concepts in metatarsal osteotomies: a remedy for metatarsalgia. Tech Foot Ankle Surg 2009;8:77–84.

4. Perry J. Gait analysis: normal and pathological function. Thorofare (NJ): Slack Inc; 1992.
5. Feibel BF, Tisdel CL, Donley BG. Lesser metatarsal osteotomies. Foot Ankle Clin 2001;6(3):473–89.
6. Barouk LS. Weil's metatarsal osteotomy in the treatment of metatarsalgia. Orthopade 1996;25(4):338–44.
7. Lau JT, Stamatis ED, Parks BG, et al. Modifications of the Weil osteotomy have no effect on plantar pressure. Clin Orthop Relat Res 2004;(421):194–8.
8. Maestro M, Besse JL, Ragusa M, et al. Forefoot morphotype study and planning method for forefoot osteotomy. Foot Ankle Clin 2003;8(4):695–710.
9. Garcia-Fernandez D, Gil-Garay E, Lora-Pablos D, et al. Comparative study of the Weil osteotomy with and without fixation. Foot Ankle Surg 2011;17(3):103–7.
10. Khurna A, Kadamabande S, James S, et al. Weil osteotomy: assessment of medium term results and predictive factors in recurrent metatarsalgia. Foot Ankle Surg 2011;17(3):150–7.
11. Trnka HJ, Gebhard C, Muhlbauer M, et al. The Weil osteotomy for treatment of dislocated lesser metatarsophalangeal joints: good outcome in 21 patients with 42 osteotomies. Acta Orthop Scand 2002;73:190–4.
12. Hart R, Janecek M, Bucek P. The Weil osteotomy in metatarsalgia. Z Orthop Ihre Grenzgeb 2003;141:590–4.
13. Vandeputte G, Dereymaeker G, Steenwerckx A, et al. The Weil osteotomy of the lesser metatarsals: a clinical and pedobarographic follow-up study. Foot Ankle Int 2000;21:370–4.
14. Jarde O, Hussenot D, Vimont E, et al. Weil's cervicocapital osteotomy for median metatarsalgia. Report of 70 cases. Acta Orthop Belg 2001;67:139–48.
15. Hofstaetter SG, Hofstaetter JG, Petroutsas JA, et al. The Weil osteotomy: a seven-year follow-up. J Bone Joint Surg Br 2005;87(11):1507–11.
16. Beech I, Rees S, Tagoe M. A retrospective review of the Weil metatarsal osteotomy for lesser metatarsal deformities: an intermediate follow-up analysis. J Foot Ankle Surg 2005;44(5):358–64.
17. Espinosa N, Brodsky JW, Maceira E. Metatarsalgia. J Am Acad Orthop Surg 2010;18:474–85.
18. Meisenbach RO. Painful anterior arch of the foot, an operation for its relief by means of raising the arch. Am J Orthop Surg 1916;14:206–11.
19. Thomas WH. Metatarsal osteotomy. Surg Clin North Am 1969;49:879–82.
20. Wolf MD. Metatarsal osteotomy for the relief of painful metatarsal callosities. J Bone Joint Surg Am 1973;55-A:1760–2.
21. Leventen E, Pearson SW. Distal metatarsal osteotomy for intractable plantar keratosis. Foot Ankle Int 1990;10:247–51.
22. Kitaoka H, Patzer GL. Chevron osteotomy of lesser metatarsals for intractable plantar callosities. J Bone Joint Surg Br 1998;80:516–8.
23. Petersen WJ, Lankes JM, Paulsen F, et al. The arterial supply of the lesser metatarsal heads: a vascular injection study in human cadavers. Foot Ankle Int 2002; 23:491–5.
24. Helal B. Metatarsal osteotomy for metatarsalgia. J Bone Joint Surg Br 1975;57-B: 187–92.
25. Helal B, Greiss M. Telescoping osteotomy for pressure metatarsalgia. J Bone Joint Surg Br 1984;66-B:213–7.
26. Winson IG, Rawlinson J, Broughton NS. Treatment of metatarsalgia by sliding distal metatarsal osteotomy. Foot Ankle 1988;9:2–6.

27. Pedowitz WJ. Distal oblique osteotomy for intractable plantar keratosis of the middle three metatarsals. Foot Ankle 1988;9:7–9.
28. Redfern DJ, Vernois J. Percutaneous surgery for metatarsalgia and the lesser toes. Foot Ankle Clin N Am 2016;21(3):527–50.
29. Henry J, Besse JL, Fessy MH, AFCP. Distal osteotomy of the lateral metatarsals: a series of 72 cases comparing the Weil osteotomy and the DMMO percutaneous osteotomy. Orthop Traumatol Surg Res 2011;97(6 Suppl):S57–65.
30. Haque S, Kakwani R, Chadwick C, et al. Outcome of minimally invasive distal metatarsal metaphyseal osteotomy (DMMO) for lesser toe metatarsalgia. Foot Ankle Int 2016;37(1):58–63.
31. Yeo NE, Loh B, Chen JY, et al. Comparison of early outcome of Weil osteotomy and distal metatarsal mini-invasive osteotomy for lesser toe metatarsalgia. J Orthop Surg (Hong Kong) 2016;24(3):350–3.
32. Redfern D, Vernois J, Legré BP. Percutaneous surgery of the forefoot. Clin Podiatr Med Surg 2015;32(3):291–332.

Treatment of Metatarsalgia with Proximal Osteotomies

Emily C. Vafek, MD, Simon Lee, MD*

KEYWORDS

- Metatarsalgia • Lesser metatarsal • Proximal osteotomy

KEY POINTS

- Proximal metatarsal osteotomies for the treatment of metatarsalgia allow for powerful deformity correction with precise control of shortening and elevation.
- Proximal metatarsal osteotomies can be technically challenging, leading to an increased risk of developing transfer lesions.
- Obtaining adequate fixation can be difficult, and patients are typically required to remain non-weight-bearing for longer periods of time.
- Many techniques have been described with little published evidence to support one over another. Generally satisfactory results have been described in several small series of patients.
- It is at the discretion of the individual surgeon to use proximal metatarsal osteotomies in select patients to reposition the metatarsal head and relieve localized forefoot pressure.

INTRODUCTION

Metatarsalgia is the general term that refers to pain in the forefoot regardless of a specific cause. Often the pain is described as being in the plantar region of the lesser metatarsal heads. Causes of metatarsalgia vary widely and can be classified into primary, secondary, and iatrogenic causes.[1] Primary causes comprise abnormalities to the anatomy of the metatarsals, especially the relationship of the metatarsal heads to one another and the rest of the foot. Relative length discrepancies, such as a longer second metatarsal or excessive plantarflexion, as seen in a cavus foot, lead to increased force in a specific area of the forefoot, which is repetitively loaded with ambulation. This overload leads to pain localized to the relatively prominent metatarsal head, and over time, patients can develop an associated plantar keratosis. Secondary

Disclosure Statement: The authors have nothing to disclose.
Department of Orthopedic Surgery, Rush University Medical Center, 1611 West Harrison Street, Suite 300, Chicago, IL 60612, USA
* Corresponding author.
E-mail address: simon.lee@rushortho.com

causes of metatarsalgia include trauma resulting in malalignment of the metatarsal and hallux rigidus, resulting in altered forefoot mechanics and transfer of pressure to the lesser metatarsals.[1] Additional examples of secondary metatarsalgia are sources of neuropathic pain, such as interdigital neuromas and tarsal tunnel syndrome, as well as osteonecrosis of the metatarsal head as seen in Freiberg disease. Iatrogenic metatarsalgia occurs following failed forefoot surgery and includes metatarsal osteotomy malposition and delayed or nonunions.[1]

CLINICAL EVALUATION

Clinical and radiographic evaluations are essential components of preoperative planning to identify and define these anatomic relationships. The patient is examined in a standing position to assess overall foot alignment. The plantar skin is inspected for the presence of diffuse or localized hyperkeratosis (**Fig. 1**), and each metatarsal head and metatarsophalangeal (MTP) joint is palpated.[2] The examiner can roll his or her index finger across the metatarsal heads with the ankle, hindfoot, and MTP joints of the lesser toes in neutral to simulate the relative position of the metatarsal heads in a flat foot stance. The same evaluation is performed with the MTP joints in dorsiflexion to simulate push-off stance and evaluate for any relative prominence.[3] Evaluation for an ankle equinus contracture should also be incorporated, because significant equinus would result in forefoot overload and may also need to be addressed. Standard weight-bearing radiographs are obtained to judge the relative length of each metatarsal as well as the overall metatarsal cascade. In addition, pedographic assessment can also elucidate plantar metatarsal prominence (**Fig. 2**). It is important to note discrepancies in relative metatarsal length and height of the metatarsal heads because the goal of surgical intervention is to restore the normal cascade and contact pressure distribution across the forefoot.

SURGICAL TREATMENT

Surgical treatment is indicated when conservative measures have failed. The goal of surgical treatment would be to reestablish the normal pressure distribution and biomechanics of the forefoot. Evaluating the whole foot and ankle to determine if

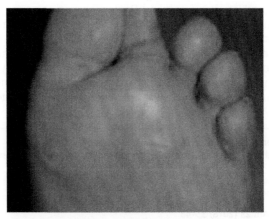

Fig. 1. Clinical photograph demonstrating localized plantar keratosis under the metatarsal heads.

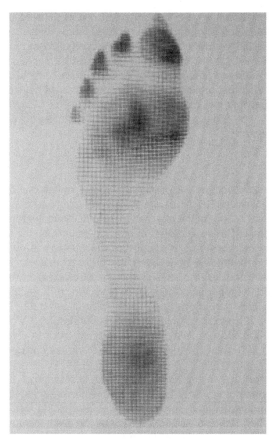

Fig. 2. Pedographic assessment; note the increased pressure under the second and third metatarsal heads.

concomitant procedures are required, that is, hallux valgus correction or gastrocnemius lengthening, is often required.

Surgical treatment of metatarsalgia can involve shortening, elevation, or both, of the metatarsal head via osteotomies through the distal, middle, or proximal aspect of the bone. Proximal osteotomies are more powerful than distal osteotomies because smaller corrections at the metatarsal base result in larger corrections at the weight-bearing metatarsal head secondary to the longer lever arm.[4] Proximal osteotomies are therefore advantageous when attempting to correct larger deformities. Other advantages of proximal osteotomies are that they are extra-articular and may minimize the risk of avascular necrosis to the metatarsal head. In addition, because they do not violate the MTP joint, there is a lower incidence of stiffness or extension drifting (floating toe) in these proximal procedures.

Although proximal osteotomies can provide powerful deformity correction, there are significant challenges involved in their implementation. Midshaft and proximal osteotomies are technically more difficult, in performing the osteotomy as well as in achieving adequate fixation. Secondary to the large corrections, proximal osteotomies are less forgiving if not optimally positioned. Overcorrection can lead to increased pressure on adjacent metatarsal heads resulting in the development of transfer lesions.[4] Proximal osteotomies are also at higher risk of delayed union or nonunion and require a longer period of immobilization and protected weight-bearing than distal osteotomies. These osteotomies typically require correction of multiple metatarsals and other deformities; as a result, careful planning of the location of the relatively extensile incisions and type of hardware placement is also critical.

A variety of midshaft and proximal metatarsal osteotomies have been described in the literature. With any of these osteotomies, the primary goal of surgery is to provide a normal distribution of pressure across the forefoot by restoring the cascade and slope of the metatarsal heads.

STEP-CUT OSTEOTOMY

In 1954, Giannestras[5] described a proximal step-cut metatarsal osteotomy for the treatment of plantar keratosis. This is primarily a shortening osteotomy. A skin incision is made on the dorsal aspect of the affected metatarsal from the tarsometatarsal joint to the midshaft distally. The dissection is carried down through the subcutaneous tissue, protecting the cutaneous nerves, and the musculature is reflected subperiosteally, exposing the metatarsal bone. A drill is used to make a series of holes to outline a 1-inch step-cut, which is subsequently completed with an osteotome (**Fig. 3**). A half-inch segment of bone is then resected from each limb of the step-cut, resulting in a half-inch shortening of the metatarsal shaft. The osteotomy is then fixed using no. 2 chromic catgut through drill holes. In the original technique, the patients were placed in a plaster of Paris walking boot in a position of plantar flexion through the MTP joints for the first 4 weeks and encouraged to ambulate as tolerated.

Giannestras[6] retrospectively reviewed the results of a series of 40 patients treated with this step-cut osteotomy. Thirty-three patients were described as having excellent results. Ten percent of patients developed transfer lesions and were reported as having good results. Two patients had recurrence of the plantar keratosis, which was attributed to insufficient shortening of the metatarsal shaft, and a third patient was deemed a failure following excision of a sesamoid for a plantar keratosis under the tibial sesamoid. This surgical procedure was determined to be technically demanding, and simpler techniques were subsequently favored.

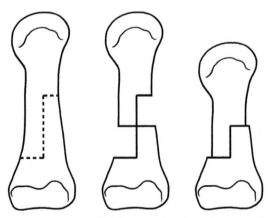

Fig. 3. The osteotomy marked out (*left*). The completed osteotomy with a portion of each limb resected (*center*). The shortened metatarsal (*right*).

MIDSHAFT SEGMENTAL OSTEOTOMY

Diaphyseal metatarsal osteotomies with resection of a cylindrical segment of bone have been described to shorten the metatarsal bone and equalize the lesser metatarsal lengths.[2] This technique allows control over the amount of bone to be resected to tailor the precise degree of shortening to the individual patient. A dorsal longitudinal skin incision is made over the midshaft of the affected metatarsal. Dissection is performed through the subcutaneous tissue to expose the periosteum of the metatarsal diaphysis. The desired segment of bone is resected using an oscillating saw with 2 parallel cuts made perpendicular to the surface of the bone (**Fig. 4**).

In 1990, Spence and colleagues[7] reported on the results of this technique used without internal fixation of the osteotomy. Eighty-nine percent of patients were described as having good to excellent results at a mean of 6 years follow-up. There were recurrent plantar keratoses in 7% of patients, and 18% developed transfer lesions. In addition, there was a 76% nonunion rate without fixation.

Galluch and colleagues[8] modified the technique to include internal fixation of the osteotomy with a 4-hole plate centered over the osteotomy and secured with 2.7-mm cortical screws (**Fig. 5**). The plate is prebent 5° to achieve compression of the plantar cortex. Further compression at the osteotomy is attained by eccentrically drilling into the proximal end of the plate holes. The resection site is packed with autogenous bone graft. Postoperatively, the patients are kept non-weight-bearing in a posterior splint for 2 weeks. From weeks 2 through 8, they are non-weight-bearing or heel-touch weight-bearing in a boot or short leg cast. Advancement to weight-bearing as tolerated is allowed at 2 months postoperatively. In the 2007 retrospective review of 126 osteotomies in 95 patients, the union rate was 99.2% within the follow-up period of 5 to 18 months, and 5 patients were reported to have developed transfer lesions. In addition, 94 of 95 patients had concomitant procedures performed, including 20 first tarsometatarsal joint fusions and 68 modified Lapidus procedures.

In 2015, DeSandis and colleagues[9] reported the results of a retrospective review of 91 osteotomies in 58 patients that had undergone segmental midshaft shortening osteotomies with internal fixation. All but 1 patient had concomitant procedures

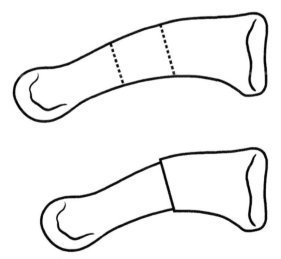

Fig. 4. The osteotomy is made as 2 parallel cuts perpendicular to the dorsal surface of the metatarsal (*top*). The shortened metatarsal (*bottom*).

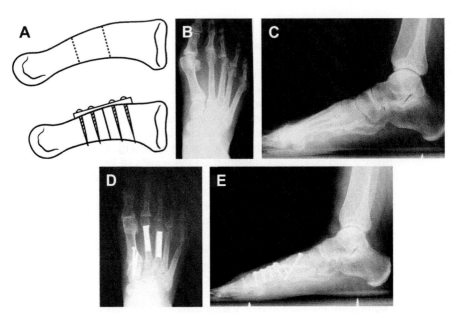

Fig. 5. (*A*) The osteotomy is made as 2 parallel cuts perpendicular to the dorsal surface of the metatarsal (*top*). The shortened metatarsal fixed with 4-hole plate and 2.7-mm screws (*bottom*). (*B*) Preoperative anteroposterior radiograph of a patient with hallux valgus and pain under the second and third metatarsal head. (*C*) Preoperative lateral radiograph. (*D*) Postoperative anteroposterior radiograph showing hallux valgus correction via first tarso-metatarsal arthrodesis and second and third metatarsal segmental shortening osteotomies restoring the cascade of the metatarsal heads. (*E*) Postoperative lateral radiograph with metatarsal heads in line with the long axis of the metatarsals. ([Radiographs provided] *Courtesy of* John Anderson, MD, Grand Rapids, MI.)

performed at the time of the metatarsal shortening osteotomy, including 11 Lapidus procedures, 13 first MTP fusions, and 15 hallux osteotomies. The mean shortening performed was 5.4 mm (2.5–8 mm). Twenty-seven osteotomies reached union by 3 months. Delayed unions were observed in 69 osteotomies, which achieved healing by 6 months postoperatively. Twenty-two osteotomies were determined to be nonunions, of which 2 reached union at 8 months, 6 reached union at 10 months, and 3 reached union by 13 months postoperatively for a final union rate of 93.4%. The investigators concluded that although midshaft segmental metatarsal osteotomies allow for precise control over the degree of metatarsal shortening and elevation, they require a prolonged period of time to achieve bony healing with a higher rate of nonunion than previously reported.

DORSAL OBLIQUE METATARSAL OSTEOTOMY

In 1991, Mann and Coughlin[10] described an oblique diaphyseal sliding osteotomy for the treatment of intractable plantar keratoses. This osteotomy is primarily a shortening osteotomy but additionally provides some degree of metatarsal head elevation. A long dorsal longitudinal incision is used to approach and expose the metatarsal shaft. If more than 5 to 6 mm of shortening is desired, the transverse metatarsal ligament is released. A transverse mark is made as an etch in the midportion of the metatarsal as a guide to the surgeon to indicate the amount of shortening achieved as the osteotomy is displaced. Using an oscillating saw, a long oblique osteotomy is made down the length of the metatarsal (**Fig. 6**). The osteotomy is oriented distal medial to proximal lateral, particularly in the second metatarsal, to avoid the artery passing between the base of the first and second metatarsals. The osteotomy is positioned to achieve the desired shortening and fixated using cerclage wires. Patients are allowed to weight-bear in a postoperative shoe if the fixation is thought to be adequate or are placed in a short-leg walking cast.

Kennedy and Deland[3] described a minor modification to this technique, preforming the osteotomy angled slightly off the direct dorsal cut. This allows for improved ease of access to temporarily pin and clamp the osteotomy as well as access during final fixation with 2 to 3 20-gauge cerclage wires. An advantage of this technique is the ability to check the desired position both clinically via direct palpation of the relative position of the metatarsal heads and radiographically to assess the cascade and make adjustments through the temporary pinning as needed. Postoperatively, patients are placed in a splint for 10 days followed by a short leg cast for 4 weeks with heel weight-bearing. Full weight-bearing is allowed at 6 weeks in a sandal. In Kennedy and Deland's series of 42 osteotomies in 32 patients, 97% (31 patients) experienced relief of plantar forefoot pain. No patients experienced transfer lesion at mean follow-up of 64 months. One patient continued to experience pain under the second metatarsal head with an associated callus, which the investigators attributed to inadequate pressure relief. The mean radiographic shortening achieved in the second and third metatarsals was 3.4 mm (1–5 mm). No patients experienced nonunion, but the time to union was determined to be slower than distal osteotomies with a mean time to radiographic union of 10 weeks (8–15 weeks). Similar to other studies on proximal osteotomies of lesser toes, a confounding variable is that 27 of the 32 patients had concomitant first metatarsal osteotomy or first tarsometatarsal fusion.

A cadaveric biomechanical study by Slovenkai and colleagues[11] compared the strength of fixation methods in dorsal oblique metatarsal osteotomies of the lesser toes. In 20 fresh frozen human cadaver bones, 10 osteotomies were fixed using crossed Kirschner wires and 10 osteotomies were fixed using a single Arbeitsgemeinschaft fur Osteosynthesefragen cortical screw via lag technique. The specimens were then subjected to load to failure testing. The investigators found the single-screw construct was significantly stiffer than the crossed wire fixation, although they noted

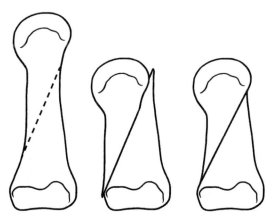

Fig. 6. The osteotomy marked out from distal medial to proximal lateral (*left*). Completed osteotomy with metatarsal slide to achieve desired shortening (*center*). The shortened metatarsal (*right*).

the mean load to failure with K-wire fixation of 20 N may be adequate for clinical application.

PROXIMAL METATARSAL OSTEOTOMY

Basal closing wedge osteotomies can be used to make powerful corrections in the dorsal or transverse plane depending on the clinical need. These osteotomies are particularly useful when a plantarflexion or adduction plane deformity is present without the need to significant shortening the metatarsal. Many variations of basal metatarsal osteotomies have been described in the literature.

Mann's technique describes a dorsal skin incision centered over the proximal half of the affected metatarsal.[12] The dissection is carried through the subcutaneous tissue with care taken to protect the cutaneous nerves down to the dorsal periosteum. The periosteum is stripped to expose the metatarsal from the base to the midshaft. The osteotomy is made at the metaphyseal flare of the base to avoid risking the saw blade impinging on the adjacent metatarsal bases. The size of the wedge removed depends on the amount of desired elevation, and a plantar cortex hinge is left intact (**Fig. 7**). The osteotomy is fixed using 22-gauge wire run through a transverse drill hole distal to the osteotomy and connecting back to a 2.7-mm screw placed in the proximal base. Patients ambulate in a postoperative shoe for 4 to 6 weeks.

A trigonometric analysis of dorsal closing wedge osteotomies in second metatarsal cadaver specimens showed the amount of elevation and shortening that can be achieved based on the width of the wedge base.[13] A 1-mm wedge corresponded to a 5-mm elevation in the metatarsal head with 5 mm gained for every 1 mm of additional bone resected so that with a base of 5 mm they demonstrated 25 mm of elevation. The lesser metatarsal bone had an absolute shortening equal to one-half the width of the base and a functional shortening of 1 to 4 mm, which was approximately equal to the width of the wedge base.

In 1983, Sclamberg and Lorenz[14] described a proximal V osteotomy for the treatment of painful plantar callosities. A V-shaped osteotomy is made at a 60° angle to

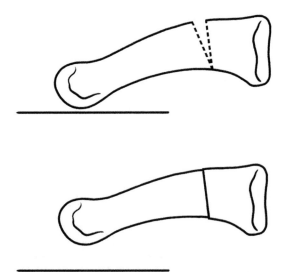

Fig. 7. The osteotomy is made as dorsal wedge (*top*) and the metatarsal head is elevated (*bottom*).

the metatarsal shaft with the apex oriented proximally toward the metatarsal base, and the plantar cortex left intact. A second V-shaped cut is made 3 to 4 mm distal to the first cut converging toward the plantar hinge, and this wedge is removed (**Fig. 8**). Upward pressure is applied to the metatarsal head to close the osteotomy with no fixation used. In their series of 41 osteotomies, the investigators described symptom relief and callosity resolution in all patients.

Barouk, Rippstein, and Toullec[15] developed a variation of a dorsal closing wedge osteotomy named the BRT osteotomy. Using a thin oscillating saw blade, a long horizontal cut is made in the proximal metaphysis directed from distal dorsal to proximal plantar (**Fig. 9**). A second cut is then made close to the first, and a segment of bone is removed with compression across the osteotomy, resulting in elevation of the metatarsal head with little shortening. Fixation is achieved with a compression screw.

In 2014, Gougoulias and Sakellariou[16] described the use of proximal closing wedge osteotomies to correct medial or lateral subluxation of lesser toes when significant plantar flexion deformity was not present. Their technique includes release of the transverse metatarsal ligament on the side of the deformity through a distal dorsal web space incision. A proximal 4-cm longitudinal incision is then made centered over the metaphysis exposing the proximal half of the affected metatarsal. The deep dissection includes elevation of the short extensor musculature off the lateral cortex. A wedge of bone is removed using a microsagittal saw, leaving a hinge intact on the far cortex (**Fig. 10**). A laminar spreader in the distal incision placed between the metatarsal heads is then used to displace the distal aspect of the metatarsal, thereby closing the gap in the proximal osteotomy gap. A 4-hole titanium locking plate is then used to fix the osteotomy. Postoperatively, patients are kept touch-down weight-bearing in a cast for 6 weeks, followed by weight-bearing in a flat stiff shoe for 6 weeks and return to unrestricted activities at 3 months. In their series of 4 patients, 3 patients had lateral deviation of the third metatarsal and 1 patient had medial deviation of the second metatarsal. At 12 months of follow-up, all 4 patients were asymptomatic and very satisfied with the outcome with maintained clinical and radiographic alignment.

Aydogan and colleagues[17] performed a comparison of proximal and distal metatarsal osteotomies in a cadaveric model in 2015. They assessed the ground reaction

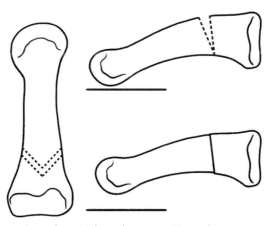

Fig. 8. The osteotomy is made as V-shaped cut at a 60° angle to metatarsal shaft (*left*). A second V-shape cut is made distally and converges on the first cut (*top*), and a wedge is removed to shorten and elevate the metatarsal (*bottom*).

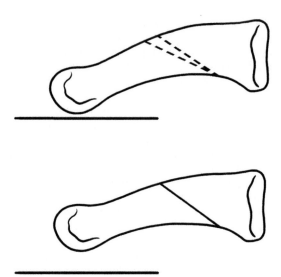

Fig. 9. The osteotomy is made as a long horizontal dorsal wedge (*top*) and the metatarsal head is elevated (*bottom*).

forces under the metatarsal heads after the osteotomies with variable static Achilles tendon loading. Their results showed that the proximal oblique osteotomy was most effective in decreasing the average and peak pressures under the second metatarsal while also increasing pressure under the first metatarsal head, indicating an effective shift in load to the first metatarsal head.

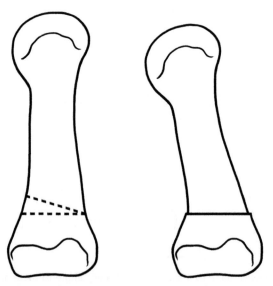

Fig. 10. The osteotomy is made as lateral wedge (*left*), and the alignment of the metatarsal is corrected in the coronal plane (*right*).

SUMMARY

Metatarsalgia is a common source of forefoot pain in patients. Careful clinical and radiographic evaluation should be performed to identify the presence of anatomic abnormities, including disruption of the normal metatarsal cascade or increased plantar prominence of the metatarsal head. Careful attention to concomitant abnormality should be undertaken because most of these patients who require a metatarsal osteotomy have additional procedures that need to be performed. Proximal metatarsal osteotomies are effective at treating metatarsalgia in patients that have failed conservative management by restoring normal metatarsal position and alleviating pressure under the metatarsal head. Proximal metatarsal osteotomies allow for powerful deformity correction with precise control of shortening and elevation, but they can be technically challenging, resulting in an increased risk of developing transfer lesions. The choice of proximal osteotomy can be determined based on whether the deformity requires shortening or elevation to achieve correction. The decision to use a proximal metatarsal osteotomy is largely based on surgeon preference because numerous techniques have been described with little supporting evidence to indicate that one procedure is significantly better than another at reliably alleviating patient symptoms while minimizing complications. Although most descriptions of proximal metatarsal osteotomies are historical in nature and rarely used, they follow well-established orthopedic concepts. Current utilization of these techniques may result in improved outcomes because of modernized fixation techniques and implants that are more specifically created for this purpose.

REFERENCES

1. Espinosa N, Brodsky JW, Maceira E. Metatarsalgia. J Am Acad Orthop Surg 2010;18(8):474–85.
2. Espinosa N, Maceira E, Myerson MS. Current concept review: metatarsalgia. Foot Ankle Int 2008;29(8):871–9.
3. Kennedy JG, Deland JT. Resolution of metatarsalgia following oblique osteotomy. Clin Orthop Relat Res 2006;453:309–13.
4. Pearce CJ, Calder JD. Metatarsalgia: proximal metatarsal osteotomies. Foot Ankle Clin 2011;16(4):597–608.
5. Giannestras NJ. Shortening of the metatarsal shaft for the correction of plantar keratosis. Clin Orthop 1954;4:225–31.
6. Giannestras NJ. Shortening of the metatarsal shaft in the treatment of plantar keratosis: an end-result study. J Bone Joint Surg Am 1958;40–A(1):61–71.
7. Spence KF, O'Connell SJ, Kenzora JE. Proximal metatarsal segmental resection: a treatment for intractable plantar keratoses. Orthopedics 1990;13(7):741–7.
8. Galluch DB, Bohay DR, Andersen JG. Midshaft metatarsal segmental osteotomy with open reduction and internal fixation. Foot Ankle Int 2007;28(2):169–74.
9. DeSandis B, Ellis SJ, Levitsky M, et al. Rate of union after segmental midshaft shortening osteotomy of the lesser metatarsals. Foot Ankle Int 2015;36(10): 1190–5.
10. Mann RA, Coughlin MJ. Intractable plantar keratosis. In: Mann RA, Coughlin MJ, editors. Video textbook of foot and ankle surgery, vol. 1. St Louis (MO): Medical Video Productions; 1991.
11. Slovenkai MP, Linehand D, McGrady L, et al. Comparison of two fixation methods of oblique lesser metatarsal osteotomies: a biomechanical study. Foot Ankle Int 1995;16(7):437–9.

12. Kaz AJ, Mann RA. Keratotic disorders of the plantar skin. In: Coughlin MJ, Saltzman CL, Anderson RB, editors. Mann's surgery of the foot and ankle. 9th edition. Philadelphia: Saunders; 2014. p. 444–7.

13. Harper MC. Dorsal closing wedge metatarsal osteotomy: a trigonometric analysis. Foot Ankle 1990;10(6):303–5.

14. Sclamberg EL, Lorenz MA. A dorsal wedge V osteotomy for painful plantar callosities. Foot Ankle 1983;4(1):30–2.

15. Barouk LS. The BRT proximal metatarsal osteotomy. In: Barouk LS, editor. Forefoot reconstruction. 2nd edition. Berlin: Springer; 2005. p. 139–54.

16. Gougoulias N, Sakellariou A. Proximal closing wedge lesser metatarsal osteotomy for metatarsophalangeal joint transverse plane realignment. Surgical technique and outcome. Foot Ankle Surg 2014;20(1):30–3.

17. Aydogan U, Moore B, Andrews S, et al. Comparison of proximal and distal oblique second metatarsal osteotomies with varying Achilles tendon tension: biomechanical study in a cadaver model. J Bone Joint Surg Am 2015;97-A(23): 1945–51.

Metatarsal Osteotomies
Complications

Veerabhadra "Babu" Reddy, MD[a,b],*

KEYWORDS

- Complications • Metatarsal • Osteotomy • Weil • Helal • Proximal • Distal

KEY POINTS

- Proximal metatarsal osteotomies can create a significant change in position of the metatarsal head and must be used judiciously to prevent transfer metatarsalgia.
- Proximal osteotomies have a higher incidence of nonunion and malunion when done without internal fixation.
- The Weil osteotomy has a high rate of union but is prone to a floating toe and recurrent metatarsalgia.

INTRODUCTION

Metatarsal osteotomies are the primary surgical tool used to deal with metatarsalgia and problems related to the lesser metatarsals. The goal of the osteotomy is to decrease the pressure underneath the respective metatarsal head during the different phases of gait. The metatarsals experience significant amounts of force during flat stance and even more so during toe-off. The first metatarsal absorbs most of the load during these phases of stance and can contribute to the disorders of the lesser metatarsal heads. This article focuses on the lesser metatarsals and the complications of the osteotomies used to address the disorders of the lesser rays.

ANATOMY

The anatomy of the lesser metatarsals is important to understand the potential complications that can arise from metatarsal osteotomies. They form a parabola that is one of the key elements to the distribution of force through the forefoot during gait. The ideal parabola is described as the second metatarsal longer than the first and greater than the third. The third metatarsal is greater than the fourth and the fourth is greater

Disclosure: The author has nothing to disclose.
[a] Department of Surgery, Texas A&M Health Science Center College of Medicine, Bryan, TX, USA; [b] Foot and Ankle Surgery Fellowship Program, Baylor University Medical Center, Dallas, 3900 Junius Street, Suite 500, Dallas, TX 75246, USA
* 6729 Kenwood Avenue, Dallas, TX 75214.
E-mail address: babu313@gmail.com

than the fifth metatarsal.[1] Although length is important, the plantar position of the metatarsal heads is also very important to determining the amount of force experienced by each head during gait. Specific foot position such as cavovarus deformities can increase or pes planovalgus deformities can decrease the declination of the metatarsals and subsequent pressure under the heads. The central metatarsals are more rigid in their position and most commonly contribute to metatarsal disorders.[2]

CLINICAL EVALUATION

Patients most commonly present with forefoot pain and overload on physical examination. Plantar tenderness that increases with gait can be localized to the offending metatarsals. The presence of intractable plantar keratosis is another sign of overload. They can be explained by the forces that travel through the forefoot during gait. As pressure is transferred from the hindfoot to the forefoot, the metatarsal heads bear an increasing load. Lesions directly underneath the metatarsal heads signify increased pressure during the stance phase of gait. A lesion distal to the metatarsal head indicates dysfunction during the toe-off phase of gait.[3] The difference between the two is important because it delineates the problem that needs to be corrected. Lesions directly underneath the metatarsal head are a sign of excess plantar pressure during stance phase and need to be alleviated by raising the metatarsal head. Lesions distal to the metatarsal heads are an indication of excessive length and correction is achieved by shortening the metatarsal length.[4]

Over the years many different types of osteotomies have been proposed and described. In general, they can be divided into 2 categories: proximal or distal. With each type of osteotomy come specific complications (**Fig. 1**).

PROXIMAL OSTEOTOMIES

Osteotomies based on the proximal aspect of the metatarsal are very powerful. A small amount of proximal resection or angulation of the metatarsal results in significant amount of shortening and elevation of the metatarsal heads. Thus preoperative planning is critical to achieve a favorable result. Traditionally the osteotomies have been described without internal fixation creating a higher incidence of nonunion and malunion (**Table 1**). (Further detail regarding the technique and images of these described osteotomies is given in Emily C. Vafek and Simon Lee's article, "Treatment of Metatarsalgia with Proximal Osteotomies," in this issue.)

STEP-CUT OSTEOTOMY

The step-cut osteotomy, described by Giannestras,[5] is a resection osteotomy and shortens the metatarsal by approximately 2.5 cm (1 inch). In the original study of 40 procedures, 37 had good or excellent outcomes. Four patients (10%) developed transfer metatarsalgia. The osteotomy is powerful, with a significant amount of shortening. Care must be taken to respect the parabola because overshortening leads to a higher incidence of transfer metatarsalgia.[5]

PROXIMAL SEGMENTAL OSTEOTOMY

The proximal segmental osteotomy resects a tubular segment of the proximal metatarsal, resulting in both shortening and elevation of the metatarsal head. Originally described without fixation, it had a very high rate of complication. Transfer metatarsalgia occurred in 18% of the study's patients and 7% of the patients experienced recurrent metatarsalgia. The most common complication, however, was the development

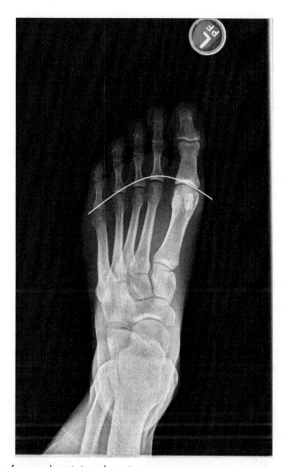

Fig. 1. Parabola of normal metatarsal anatomy.

of a nonunion, which happened in 76% of the patients. At 6 months 75.8% of osteotomies still had not developed union. At 13 months, 85 of 91 osteotomies had healed. Ultimately there was only a 6.6% nonunion rate. Although it was not proved to be statistically significant, there was an increased trend toward delayed healing in feet that required more than 1 metatarsal osteotomy.[6] Modifying this osteotomy with the addition of internal fixation significantly reduces the rate of nonunion. Galluch and colleagues[7] used a plate to stabilize the osteotomy, increasing the rate of union to

Table 1 Complications of proximal osteotomies	
Proximal Osteotomy	**Common Complications**
Step-cut osteotomy	Excessive shortening
Proximal segmental osteotomy	Nonunion when done without fixation
Oblique diaphyseal metatarsal osteotomy	Delayed union
Barouk–Rippstein–Toullec (BRT) osteotomy	Excessive dorsiflexion and transfer metatarsalgia

99.2%. The postoperative course, however, requires the patients to be non–weight bearing for 2 months (**Fig. 2**).

OBLIQUE DIAPHYSEAL METATARSAL OSTEOTOMY

The oblique diaphyseal osteotomy uses an oblique cut through the diaphysis to allow shortening and elevation of the metatarsal. The cut is made in a vertical plane starting distal lateral and extending through the entire metatarsal shaft to exit proximal and medial. The metatarsal is then allowed to slide on itself, resulting in shortening and elevation of the metatarsal head. In the technique described by Kennedy and Deland,[8] special attention was paid to the plantar prominence of the metatarsal head. The obliquity of the osteotomy allows for dorsal translation of the metatarsal head in order to decrease plantar pressure. Inadequate dorsiflexion of the metatarsal head results in recurrent metatarsalgia, or excessive dorsal translation of the metatarsal head can result in transfer metatarsalgia. In their study, 31 of 32 patients had complete resolution of metatarsalgia. The diaphyseal osteotomy did have increased time to healing, with a mean of 10 weeks to radiographic union.[8]

PROXIMAL V OSTEOTOMY

The proximal V osteotomy is traditionally performed without any internal fixation. This osteotomy relies on preserving the plantar cortex for stability. A dorsal wedge of bone is resected with either a rongeur or sagittal saw. Plantar pressure is then applied to close the osteotomy. The patient is asked to immediately weight bear to keep the osteotomy closed and to achieve the appropriate amount of dorsiflexion relative to

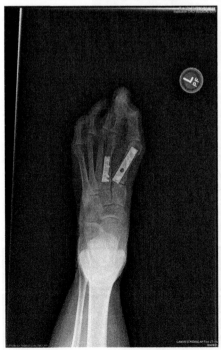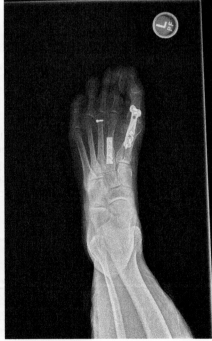

Fig. 2. Radiograph of excessive shortening with proximal segmental osteotomy.

the pressure that is felt during weight bearing. Sclamberg and Lorenz[9] reported no complications in 41 patients.

BAROUK–RIPPSTEIN–TOULLEC OSTEOTOMY

This is an oblique basal osteotomy of the metatarsal. It is primarily used to elevate the metatarsal head to relieve metatarsalgia through a proximal osteotomy performed at a 60° angle to the longitudinal axis of the metatarsal with an intact plantar hinge. It creates a stable osteotomy that allows patients to weight bear 2 weeks postoperatively. Care must be taken to avoid excessive dorsiflexion and transfer metatarsalgia.[10]

DISTAL METATARSAL OSTEOTOMIES

Distal metatarsal osteotomies have inherent advantages compared with proximal osteotomies. Metatarsal osteotomies are commonly done in combination with procedures on the lesser toes, allowing both procedures to be done through a smaller incision. The distal metatarsal also provides a more vascular region of bone in the metaphyseal area to allow better healing of the osteotomy. This wider metaphyseal region provides a more stable surface to further increase the rate of healing. However, these advantages come with complications that are specific to the distal osteotomy (**Table 2**) (Further details regarding the technique and images of these described osteotomies are given in David Redfern's article, "Treatment of Metatarsalgia with Distal Osteotomies," in this issue.)

DISTAL CHEVRON OSTEOTOMY

In a study of the distal chevron osteotomy, 16 of 21 feet had good results without any nonunions. Transfer metatarsalgia was found in 3 of the 21 feet. The osteotomy is elevated about 2 to 3 mm and shortened on average of 2.6 mm.[9] A study of the distal chevron osteotomy stabilized by a T plate showed a 3% rate of nonunion, 6% hypertrophic nonunion, and 3% floating toe.[11]

DISTAL OBLIQUE OSTEOTOMY

Originally described by Helal[12] in 1975, the Helal osteotomy is a distal oblique osteotomy that resulted in an 88% good to excellent result. A cut is made at an angle of 45° to the metatarsal shaft from proximal dorsal to distal plantar. The metatarsal head is then loosened with an osteotome and allowed to translate dorsally and proximally. Traditionally, no fixation is used to stabilize the osteotomy.[12] Multiple studies examined the efficacy of the Helal osteotomy and were unable to replicate the original data. The complications are primarily caused by the lack of internal fixation and

Table 2 Complications of distal metatarsal osteotomies	
Distal Osteotomy	**Complication**
Helal osteotomy	Malunion resulting in transfer metatarsalgia Nonunion of 7%–15%
Weil osteotomy	Arthrofibrosis and stiffness Floating toe Recurrent metatarsalgia with inadequate dorsal translation
Distal chevron osteotomy	Difficult to shorten the metatarsal

stabilization of the osteotomy. The rate of nonunion ranges from 7% to 15% in the literature.[13–16] The incidence of malunion, which manifests as transfer metatarsalgia and continued pain, varies but overall is at an unacceptably high level. Winson and colleagues[14] showed that 40% of patients had residual plantar prominence and pain after a Helal osteotomy. Trnka and colleagues[16] published results of 19 malunions and 8 nonunions in 96 patients. At 10 years, one study showed that 50% of patients still had pain.[16] The addition of internal fixation decreased the rate of nonunion and malunion. Cheng and colleagues[17] published results in which the addition of fixation decreased the rate of malunion to 1 in 22 patients.

WEIL OSTEOTOMY

The Weil osteotomy has been the workhorse procedure for metatarsalgia and metatarsal disorders for many years. It is a very stable osteotomy done through the distal metatarsal head and metaphyseal bone. The nonunion rate reported in the literature is very low. A literature review showed that, out of 1131 osteotomies, there was a 3% nonunion rate. The combination of internal fixation with the stable plane of the osteotomy allows this low rate of nonunion.[18]

The Weil osteotomy, however, is intraarticular because the saw cut is done within the dorsal aspect of the metatarsal head. This procedure violates the articular cartilage and leads to a significant amount of stiffness within the metatarsal phalangeal joint. In addition to violating the articular cartilage with the osteotomy, the exposure of the metatarsophalangeal joint requires opening the capsule. The combination of the exposure and osteotomy leads to arthrofibrosis and stiffness of the joint. Examination of the range of motion 7 years after osteotomy showed 48% of joints with a moderate restriction in range of motion (30°–75°) and 20% with a severe restriction in range of motion (<30°).[19]

Although it is a stable osteotomy, the Weil osteotomy can result in transfer metatarsalgia, which is usually secondary to inadequate attention paid to the relative length of the adjacent metatarsals. A study reviewing the amount of proximal shift that increased the rate of transfer lesions found that greater than 4.5 mm of proximal shift resulted in a higher incidence of transfer lesions. The optimal amount of shortening was between 3 and 4.5 mm.[20]

A review of the literature showed transfer lesions in between 0% and 18.8% of patients. Overall, a 7% incidence of transfer lesions was found with the Weil osteotomy.[18]

Recurrent metatarsalgia is also a known complication of the Weil osteotomy. The single oblique cut when translated proximally increases the amount of plantar displacement of the metatarsal head and in turn leads to the approximately 15% recurrence rate of metatarsalgia after the Weil osteotomy.[18] To examine the position of the metatarsal head in the transverse plain, a radiograph called the metatarsal skyline view was used to assess the position of the metatarsal head after the osteotomy relative to the adjacent metatarsal heads. Of the 61 patients in the study, 55 patients had a good to excellent result and 6 had a poor result. Those with the poor result had an increased incidence of plantar prominence on the radiographic skyline view **(Fig. 3)**.[21]

Attention must also be paid to the angle of the cut. Originally described to be parallel to the weight-bearing surface of the foot, this ideal cut is difficult to achieve. An increase in angulation of the cut relative to the metatarsal results in a decreased amount of shortening and increased amount of plantar pressure underneath the metatarsal head.

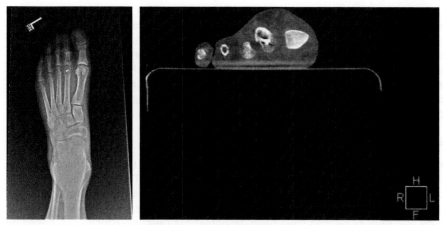

Fig. 3. Excessive dorsal translation after Weil osteotomy.

To prevent the plantar displacement of the metatarsal head with proximal shortening of the Weil osteotomy, a wedge of bone is resected from the osteotomy to add dorsal translation. Melamed and colleagues[22] studied the osteotomy on saw bones and showed that resecting a dorsal wedge eliminates the plantar translation that occurs with the proximal shift. The wedge is created by a second cut parallel to the initial osteotomy.

An intraoperative radiograph and palpation of the plantar surface of the foot can help determine whether an adequate amount of bone was resected to decrease the plantar prominence of the metatarsal head.

The most common complication following the Weil osteotomy is the floating toe. The proximal and plantar translation of the metatarsal head changes the axis of rotation of the metatarsal phalangeal joint relative to the intrinsic muscles of the foot. By moving the metatarsal head plantarly, the intrinsics change from creating a plantar flexion force to more of a dorsiflexion force because the vector is now dorsal to the axis of rotation. The literature shows between 20% and 36% incidence of floating toe after a Weil osteotomy.[18,23]

Migues and colleagues[24] showed a correlation between the incidence of a floating toe and a proximal interphalangeal joint (PIP) arthroplasty done in conjunction with the metatarsal osteotomy. Fifty percent of the toes that had PIP arthroplasty developed a floating toe, whereas only 15% of those without a PIP arthroplasty developed a floating toe.

Although the removal of a wedge of bone decreases the plantar translation of the metatarsal head and theoretically preserves the axis of rotation and position of the intrinsic musculature, the literature shows no significant decrease in the rate of floating toes when the wedge resection is added to the procedure. Another theory regarding development of a floating toe is the disruption of the windlass mechanism. The tension generated by the plantar plate and metatarsophalangeal joint with toe-off allows the stable hinge motion of the joint. The attenuation of the plantar plate created by a chronic subluxed metatarsophalangeal joint or increased pressure underneath the metatarsal head leads to laxity of the plantar plate. This laxity is increased when combined with a shortening osteotomy of the metatarsal head. Thus, the increased laxity of the poor-quality tissue may lead to the high incidence of floating toes.[18]

The floating toe is a common complication of the Weil osteotomy but has little impact on the patients' overall function and satisfaction. The metatarsalgia is usually resolved, allowing improvement in pain and functional scores. Gregg and colleagues[25] combined a metatarsal osteotomy with an extensor digitorum longus lengthening and plantar plate reconstruction, resulting in a 6% incidence a floating toe. The flexor to extensor tendon transfer is also used to help stabilize the joint and decrease the incidence of the floating toe. Many surgeons also pin the joint in plantar flexion to allow the plantar plate and collateral ligaments to stabilize the joint.

SUMMARY

Metatarsal osteotomies, proximal and distal, are intended to decrease the pressure under the metatarsal head to improve function and gait. They can also be used in conjunction with procedures on the lesser toes to correct subluxation/dislocation of the metatarsophalangeal joint and hammer toe deformities. The different complications and their incidences have been described but definitive conclusions based on the literature are hard to draw. From the literature, internal fixation for both proximal and distal osteotomies reduces the rate of nonunion or malunion. Proximal osteotomies are powerful and must be done prudently to avoid excessive dorsiflexion and transfer metatarsalgia.

With regard to distal osteotomies, the Helal osteotomy has a higher rate of complication than the Weil osteotomy. The Weil osteotomy with internal fixation achieves a more reproducible and reliable correction of metatarsalgia. The addition of a wedge resection decreases the plantar translation of the head and reduces the incidence of recurrent metatarsalgia. The high incidence of the floating toe is most likely secondary to multiple factors: the shortening of the ray and laxity of the plantar plate and extrinsic musculature, the change in the axis of rotation of the metatarsophalangeal joint. This complication, however, has little impact on the overall function and satisfaction of the patient.

REFERENCES

1. Maestro M, Besse JL, Ragusa M, et al. Forefoot morphotype study and planning method for forefoot osteotomy. Foot Ankle Clin 2003;8:695–710.
2. Feibel JB, Tisdel CL, Donley BG. Lesser metatarsal osteotomies. Foot Ankle Clin 2001;6:473–89.
3. Espinosa N, Brodsky JW, Maceira E. Metatarsalgia. J Am Acad Orthop Surg 2010;18:474–85.
4. Schuh R, Trnka HJ. Metatarsalgia: distal metatarsal osteotomies. Foot Ankle Clin 2011;16(4):583–95.
5. Giannestras NJ. Shortening of the metatarsal shaft in the treatment of plantar keratosis: an end-result study. Foot Ankle Int 1995;16:529–34.
6. Spence KF, O'Connell SJ, Kenzora JE. Proximal metatarsal segmental resection: a treatment for intractable plantar keratoses. Orthopedics 1990;13(7):741–7.
7. Galluch DB, Bohay DR, Anderson JG. Midshaft metatarsal segmental osteotomy with open reduction and internal fixation. Foot Ankle Int 2007;28(2):169–74.
8. Kennedy JG, Deland JT. Resolution of metatarsalgia following oblique osteotomy. Clin Orthop Relat Res 2006;453:309–13.
9. Sclamberg EL, Lorenz MA. A dorsal wedge V osteotomy for painful plantar callosities. Foot Ankle 1983;4(1):30–2.
10. Barouk LS. Forefoot reconstruction. Paris: Springer; 2003. p. 117, 109–48, 168–72.

11. Herzog JL, Goforth WD, Stone PA, et al. A modified fixation technique for a decompression shortening osteotomy: a retrospective analysis. J Foot Ankle Surg 2014;53(2):131–6.
12. Helal B. Metatarsal osteotomy for metatarsalgia. J Bone Joint Surg Br 1975;57: 187–92.
13. Pedowitz WJ. Distal oblique osteotomy for intractable plantar keratosis of the middle three metatarsals. Foot Ankle Int 1988;9:7–9.
14. Winson IG, Rawlinson J, Broughton NS. Treatment of metatarsalgia by sliding distal metatarsal osteotomy. Foot Ankle 1988;9:2–6.
15. Idusuyi OB, Kitaoka HG, Patzer GL. Oblique metatarsal osteotomy for intractable plantar keratosis: 10-year follow-up. Foot Ankle Int 1988;19:351–5.
16. Trnka HJ, Kabon B, Zehl R, et al. Current topics in international foot and ankle surgery: Helal metatarsal osteotomy for the treatment of metatarsalgia: a critical analysis of results. Orthopedics 1995;19:457–61.
17. Cheng YM, Lin SY, Wu CK, et al. Oblique sliding metatarsal osteotomy for pressure metatarsalgia. J Med Sci 1992;8:403–11.
18. Highlander P, VonHerbulis E, Gonzalez A, et al. Complications of the Weil osteotomy. Foot Ankle Spec 2011;4(3):165–70.
19. Hofstaetter SG, Hofstaetter JG, Petroutsas JA, et al. The Weil osteotomy: a seven-year follow up. J Bone Joint Surg Br 2005;87(11):1507–11.
20. Dreeben SM, Noble PC, Hammerman S, et al. Metatarsal osteotomy for primary metatarsalgia: radiographic and pedobarographic study. Foot Ankle Int 1989;9: 214–8.
21. Khurana A, Kadamabande S, James S, et al. Weil osteotomy: assessment of medium term results and predictive factors in recurrent metatarsalgia. J Foot Ankle Surg 2011;17(3):150–7.
22. Melamed EA, Schon LC, Myerson MS, et al. Two modifications of the Weil osteotomy: analysis on sawbone models. Foot Ankle Int 2002;23(5):400–5.
23. O'Kane C, Kilmartin TE. The surgical management of central metatarsalgia. Foot Ankle Int 2002;23(5):415–9.
24. Migues A, Slullitel G, Bilbao F, et al. Floating-toe deformity as a complication of the Weil osteotomy. Foot Ankle Int 2004;25(9):609–13.
25. Gregg J, Silberstein M, Clark C, et al. Plantar plate repair and Weil osteotomy for metatarsophalangeal joint instability. Foot Ankle Surg 2007;13:116–21.

Gastrocnemius Recession for Metatarsalgia

Rose E. Cortina, MD*, Brandon L. Morris, MD, Bryan G. Vopat, MD

KEYWORDS

- Strayer • Gastrocnemius recession • Endoscopic gastrocnemius recession
- Metatarsalgia

KEY POINTS

- Metatarsalgia is a common cause of forefoot pain with various causes.
- Isolated gastrocnemius contracture is one contributor of forefoot pain that is diagnosed with use of the Silfverskiold test.
- Patients with a positive Silfverskiold test that have failed nonoperative management a gastrocnemius lengthening is a treatment option to offload the forefoot.
- Gastrocnemius lengthening in patients with isolated gastrocnemius contracture is performed either open or endoscopic.

INTRODUCTION

Metatarsalgia, also known as metatarsal pain, represents one of most frequently cited causes of pain in patients seeking foot care.[1,2] In a general sense, metatarsalgia may refer to a variety of painful conditions arising from the forefoot; however, the term also exists as a discrete diagnosis to describe plantar forefoot pain beneath the second, third, and fourth metatarsal heads.[2–4] The causes of metatarsalgia vary greatly and may arise from primary causes or result secondary to pathologic conditions arising from other locations within the foot and ankle. Identifying the exact location of metatarsalgia pain generators may be simple, or complex, as the cause of pain may involve the hindfoot, ankle, or even leg.[2] Treatment of metatarsalgia varies widely owing to the numerous causes of the condition. Management may involve nonoperative measures, such as orthotic use or physical therapy. More severe cases may require surgical intervention to address bony foot deformity, soft tissue imbalance, or a compressive neuropathy. Appropriate treatment of metatarsalgia requires an individualized approach to treatment derived from a thorough history and meticulous physical examination.

Disclosure Statement: The authors have nothing to disclose.
Department of Orthopedic surgery, University of Kansas Medical Center, 3901 Rainbow Boulevard, Kansas City, KS 66160, USA
* Corresponding author.
E-mail address: rcortina@kumc.edu

Foot Ankle Clin N Am 23 (2018) 57–68
https://doi.org/10.1016/j.fcl.2017.09.006
1083-7515/18/© 2017 Elsevier Inc. All rights reserved.

foot.theclinics.com

Prior investigators have classified metatarsalgia into 3 broad groups: primary, secondary, and iatrogenic.[2]

Primary Metatarsalgia

Primary metatarsalgia consists of intrinsic forefoot abnormalities related to the metatarsal anatomy. Metatarsal deformity contributes to overload of adjacent metatarsals, thus, causing pain. Conditions involving primary metatarsalgia include metatarsal length discrepancy, excessive metatarsal plantar flexion, first ray insufficiency, forefoot equinus, and metatarsal head abnormality.

Secondary Metatarsalgia

Secondary metatarsalgia refers to extrinsic pathology that indirectly overloads the second to fourth metatarsal heads. These conditions include posttraumatic metatarsal malalignment resulting from malunion or nonunion, lesser metatarsal overload resulting from hallux rigidus or metatarsal phalangeal joint instability, neuropathic pain caused by an interdigital neuroma or tarsal tunnel syndrome, and Freiberg infarction.

Iatrogenic Metatarsalgia

Iatrogenic metatarsalgia may occur from various sources. Iatrogenic causes of metatarsalgia include malunion after metatarsal osteotomy or resection of the metatarsal head. One frequent cause of iatrogenic metatarsalgia is shortening of the second metatarsal due to nonunion, fracture deformity, or an incorrectly selected lesser metatarsal osteotomy.[2]

Isolated gastrocnemius contracture mimicking primary metatarsalgia has been shown to cause increased pressure and overload of the forefoot during the gait leading to metatarsal pain.[5–9] The prevalence of isolated gastrocnemius contracture varies. DiGiovanni and colleagues[9] reported 75% of patients in a cohort of 34 patients with symptomatic foot and ankle pathology were found to have an isolated gastrocnemius contracture. Hill[10] studied 209 consecutive new patients presenting with primary foot complaints and found that 176 (96.5%) demonstrated restricted ankle dorsiflexion requiring compensation during gait.

In the setting of an isolated gastrocnemius contracture, foot biomechanics compensate for decreased ankle dorsiflexion by increased recruitment of extensor digitorum longus and extensor halluces longus during the swing phase of the gait. This muscle recruitment shifts weight-bearing pressure from the hindfoot to the forefoot.[5,11] Additionally, overextension of the metatarsal phalangeal joints uncovers the metatarsal head, which applies more direct plantar force on the metatarsal head. Previous studies have demonstrated a higher prevalence of gastrocnemius shortening in patients with foot pain in comparison with the general population.[5,7,9] Treatment directed at lengthening the gastrocnemius or gastrocnemius/soleus complex through nonsurgical or surgical techniques serves to reduce the pressure at the forefoot.

CLINICAL EXAMINATION

An accurate diagnosis of metatarsalgia requires a thorough examination of the foot, ankle, and leg to identify the mechanism by which the metatarsals experience weight-bearing overload. One key method with which to evaluate patients is to determine if patients have an equinus contracture. It is paramount that the subtalar joint is locked in inversion while dorsiflexing the ankle to prevent patients from appearing to have more dorsiflexion through the subtalar joint. The subtalar joint's oblique axis of rotation causes the appearance of dorsiflexion when the joint is everted (**Fig. 1**). The

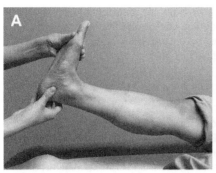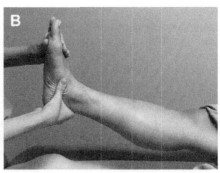

Fig. 1. Examination of the ankle. (*A*) Hindfoot eversion causing pseudodorsiflexion when the talonavicular joint is not reduced. (*B*) Reduced talonavicular joint locks the midfoot and hindfoot in neutral showing an equinus contracture in the same patient.

average ankle dorsiflexion varies among patients with and without foot and ankle pathology. Jastifer and Marston[12] measured ankle dorsiflexion in 66 consecutive patients with foot and ankle complaints and compared their ankle dorsiflexion values with an equal-numbered control group. They found a mean ankle dorsiflexion of 11.6° in the foot- and ankle-pain groups compared with a mean of 17.2° in the control group (*P*<.0001). These values are similar to those previously reported by DiGiovanni and colleagues[9] in 2002 of 13.1° average ankle dorsiflexion in control-group patients. Having identified a pathologic deficit in ankle dorsiflexion, the clinician must then determine whether the contracture exists because of gastrocnemius-soleus complex contracture or an isolated gastrocnemius contracture. The Silfverskiold test enables the clinical examiner to differentiate between the two underlying intrinsic causes of equinus contracture. To perform the Silfverskiold test, patients lie supine and the clinician evaluates ankle dorsiflexion first with the ipsilateral knee extended and then with the knee flexed. During the test, the foot is held in an inverted position to prevent dorsiflexion through the subtalar joint. The Silfverskiold test reveals an isolated gastrocnemius contracture when patients are unable to reach neutral ankle dorsiflexion with the knee extended but then ankle dorsiflexion increases 15° to 20° with the knee flexed.[13] Silfverskiold[14] defined gastrocnemius contracture as ankle dorsiflexion of less than 5° with the knee extended that improves to 10° of ankle dorsiflexion with the knee flexed[14,15] (**Fig. 2**). If ankle dorsiflexion remains unchanged with the knee

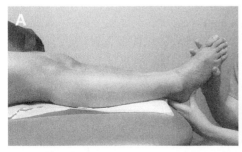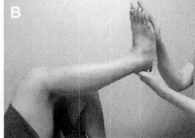

Fig. 2. Silfverskiold test in a patient with an isolated gastrocnemius contracture. (*A*) Limited ankle dorsiflexion with the knee extended. (*B*) Improved ankle dorsiflexion with the knee flexed to 90°.

flexed as compared with the knee extended, then both the gastrocnemius muscle and soleus muscle or Achilles contribute to the equinus deformity.[14] Patients with a secondary metatarsalgia whose Silfverskiold test reveals an equinus contracture due to gastrocnemius tightness and no other identifiable cause of pain may benefit from a gastrocnemius release.

NONOPERATIVE TREATMENT

The first-line treatment of metatarsalgia secondary to a gastrocnemius contracture should consist of nonoperative measures. Evidence regarding the efficacy of these nonoperative measures varies greatly; however, physical therapy and shoe modification, or a combination of the two approaches, represent appropriate initial treatment modalities.

Given the high prevalence of equinus contracture within the general population, nonoperative intervention to address secondary metatarsalgia should be initially prescribed. Physical therapy focuses on stretching posterior calf structures to improve ankle dorsiflexion, thereby restoring normal gait mechanics and reducing forefoot pressure placed on the metatarsals. Lengthening the triceps surae can lead to decreased pressure experienced at the forefoot.[1,2,16,17] Active stretching can be done by placing the midfoot on a step with the knee in extension followed by lowering the heel as much as possible and maintaining this position for 10 seconds (**Fig. 3**). Patients are typically advised to perform 20 consecutive stretches 3 times daily, which amounts to roughly 20 minutes daily. Another type of gastrocnemius stretch may be done passively, whereby patients stand on an inclined board, which positions the ankle in dorsiflexion. A randomized controlled trial of a 6-week stretching program has shown to increase ankle dorsiflexion and passive tendon length.

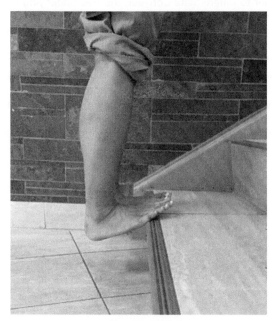

Fig. 3. Active gastrocnemius exercise whereby the midfoot is on a step with the knee in extension followed by lowering the heel as much as possible and maintaining this position for 10 seconds.

Whether stretching interventions effectively increase joint mobility and muscle excursion remains controversial. One systematic review examined 13 studies and found that regular stretching of healthy tissues without contracture increased joint range of motion by 8° on average, with gains lasting for more than 1 day after cessation of stretching. The effects of stretching were found to be greatest in muscle groups with limited extensibility.[18] Radford and colleagues[19] conducted a meta-analysis of randomized controlled trials comparing static calf muscle stretching with no stretching and found that ankle dorsiflexion increased on average 2.07° stretching less than 15 minutes ($P<.001$), 3.03° after stretching 15 to 30 minutes ($P = .03$), and 2.49° after stretching more than 30 minutes ($P = .04$).[19,20] These results imply a small yet statistically significant increase in ankle dorsiflexion after performing posterior calf stretching exercises. Knowing, however, that an efficient gait requires 5° to 18° of ankle dorsiflexion, the gains acquired through stretching interventions may simply be too small to effectively address metatarsalgia secondary to isolated gastrocnemius contracture.[13,21] In these patients, surgical intervention may be indicated.

Shoe modification or orthotic inserts consists of wide toe boxes, a well-cushioned sole, decreased heel height, the use of a metatarsal bar, or a rocker bottom sole to ease push-off pressure and facilitate gait propulsion. Metatarsal bars help redistribute plantar pressure experienced in the forefoot. A prospective study has shown that a metatarsal bar placed proximal to the metatarsal head can help alleviate pressure and pain over the forefoot.[2,22,23]

SURGICAL DECISION-MAKING PRINCIPLES

Surgical lengthening of the triceps surae complex or the gastrocnemius in isolation is indicated once nonoperative treatment modalities have failed to provide patients with sufficient relief of metatarsalgia symptoms when the cause is from a contracted gastrocnemius. Surgical lengthening of posterior leg soft tissues is performed to reduce plantar forces experienced on the metatarsals. Operative techniques vary and include open and endoscopic surgical approaches. The sural nerve is at risk during the surgical intervention; patients may also experience decreased ankle plantar flexion strength, and some patients may complain of cosmesis because of a change in the shape of the calf postoperatively.[24]

Key to successful surgical intervention is thorough anatomic understanding of the structures that will be encountered during surgery. Such mastery allows for safe and efficient surgery and reduces the risk of iatrogenic complications. The gastrocnemius, soleus, and plantaris muscles comprise the superficial posterior compartment of the leg. Of the 3, the gastrocnemius is the largest and most superficial muscle. Crossing the knee, ankle, and subtalar joints, the gastrocnemius is a biarticular muscle, with 2 heads that originate on the medial and lateral femoral condyles. These muscle heads then traverse distally joining at the midline. The combined gastrocnemius muscle belly continues down the leg to where the gastrocnemius merges with the soleus muscle to form the Achilles tendon. The soleus muscle originates from the posterior aspect of the tibia, fibula, and the interosseous membrane, coursing deep to the gastrocnemius. Before forming the Achilles tendon, both the gastrocnemius and the soleus form an aponeurosis transitioning into individual tendons that glide independently proximal to their confluence at the Achilles tendon. The gastrocnemius tendon inserts into the Achilles an average of 18 mm from the visible indentation on the calf and an average of 159 mm proximal to the Achilles insertion onto the calcaneus.[25] Structures at risk during surgical lengthening of the gastrocnemius soleus complex include the sural nerve. Formed by the medial sural cutaneous nerve and the lateral sural cutaneous nerve, the sural nerve begins at the distal third of the gastrocnemius and descends along the posterolateral aspect of the leg. Pinney and colleagues[25] reviewed the surgical anatomy of the Strayer procedure and found that at the level of surgical release, the sural nerve is found on average 46 mm from the medial border of the gastrocnemius tendon. In 57.5% of the Strayer procedures performed, the sural nerve was identified deep to the fascia at the surgical site located at the insertion point of the gastrocnemius tendon into the Achilles tendon.[25] Careful placement of the surgical incision must be taken to prevent sural nerve injury during surgical lengthening of the gastrocnemius soleus complex.

When proceeding with surgical treatment of metatarsalgia secondary to equinus contracture, surgeons must first identify which structure to surgically lengthen based on their physical examination of patients, revealing either an isolated gastrocnemius contracture or a contracture of the gastrocnemius-soleus complex.

Open Surgical Treatment

Multiple surgical techniques have been described to release an isolated gastrocnemius contracture. Surgical techniques vary in their anatomic location and method of release. Gastrocnemius tendon release was initially described by Vulpius[26] in 1913 and later further elaborated by Strayer[27] in 1950. Strayer described an open surgical technique using a posterior or posteromedial incision (the authors prefer a posteromedial incision) at the level of the musculotendinous junction. This anatomic landmark can be found just distal to the gastrocnemius indentation on the posterior calf. This technique is performed with patients in either a supine or prone position. Dissection is carried down to the posterior fascia taking care to identify and preserve the sural cutaneous nerve, which lies deep to the posterior gastrocnemius fascia. At this level, the sural nerve may be adherent to either the fascia or the muscle belly. The fascia is incised in line with the skin incision, and the gastrocnemius tendon is isolated from the underlying soleus. This isolation can be done by placing your finger between the gastrocnemius and the soleus allowing easy visualization of the gastrocnemius tendon (**Fig. 4**A). The distal end of the gastrocnemius aponeurosis is then cut sharply either with a knife or scissors (**Fig. 4**B). Strayer's[27] original description called for the gastrocnemius fascia to be sutured to the underlying soleus fascia in its lengthened position; however, more recent modifications omit this step.[25,27] The gastrocnemius is then lengthened by placing constant dorsiflexion on the foot until appropriate dorsiflexion is achieved. It is the authors' preference to perform this procedure in this way without repairing the fascia to the soleus. The subcutaneous tissue is closed with dissolvable suture followed by either a running nylon or staples.

Additional open gastrocnemius surgical lengthening includes the medial proximal gastrocnemius release and the Baumann procedure. The medial proximal gastrocnemius release was developed to reduce the risk of sural nerve injury and improve surgical site cosmesis.[24,25] To perform the proximal gastrocnemius release, patients are positioned prone and a 2- to 3-cm transverse incision along the Langer lines on the medial portion of the popliteal flexion crease is made. Once exposed, the medial head of the gastrocnemius muscle fibers are released off the tibia, taking care to distinguish the gastrocnemius from the neighboring structures.[13] Baumann[28] also described a method to surgically lengthen the gastrocnemius muscle. With patients supine, a medial longitudinal incision is made at the midcalf level and proximal to the release location at the musculotendinous junction described by Strayer.[27] After the incision is made, the crural fascia is identified as well as the greater saphenous vein and saphenous nerve. Next, after incising the crural fascia, the gastrocnemius muscle belly is bluntly dissected away from the soleus muscle belly. At this

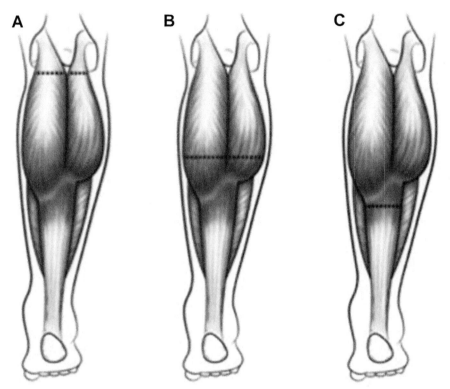

Fig. 4. The different location sites of the release of the gastrocnemius are demonstrated in a proximal gastrocnemius release (*A*), a Baumann release (*B*), and a Strayer/Vulpius release (*C*).

intermuscular level, the plantaris is encountered and transected. To place tension along the gastrocnemius, the ankle is then dorsiflexed and a transverse incision is then made on the deep undersurface of the gastrocnemius muscle. Incisions in this tendinous portion are made until the desired dorsiflexion is obtained.[29,30] The Vulpius release entails transection of the gastrocnemius aponeurosis posteriorly distal to the middle of the leg without dissection of the gastrocnemius aponeurosis from the underlying soleus muscle (**Fig. 4**C). A diagram of the relative anatomic locations of each surgical lengthening technique may be found in **Fig. 5**.[31]

Endoscopic Treatment

An alternative to open surgical techniques, endoscopic gastrocnemius recession was initially developed to reduce injury to the soleus muscle fibers when isolating gastrocnemius fibers. The endoscopic technique uses 2 incisions, one each on the medial and lateral side of the gastrocnemius musculotendinous junction. Through blunt dissection, the fascia is approached and a slotted cannula is inserted into the medial incision, followed by a 4-mm endoscope. The cannula should be deep to the crural fascia but superficial to the gastrocnemius aponeurosis (**Fig. 6**A). Cotton swabs may be used to clear away fatty tissue to improve visualization. The gastrocnemius aponeurosis and sural nerve are then identified with a 30° endoscopic camera; with the ankle dorsiflexed, the gastrocnemius is incised (**Fig. 6**B).[29,32,33]

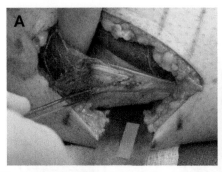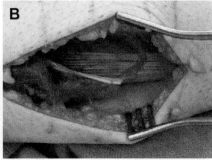

Fig. 5. Strayer release: (*A*) Isolation of the gastrocnemius from the gastrosoleus complex to allow direct visualization before release. (*B*) Completed gastrocnemius recession. (*From* Abdulmassih S, Phisitkul P, Femino J, et al. Triceps surae contracture: implications for foot and ankle surgery. J Am Acad Orthop Surg 2013;21:403; with permission.)

POSTOPERATIVE PROTOCOL

Patients start non–weight bearing in a splint in maximum dorsiflexion for 2 weeks until the incision heals. At 2 weeks postoperatively, patients may bear weight with a controlled ankle motion (CAM) boot as needed. Calf stretches and isometric exercises can also begin at this time. During the 2- to 4-week postoperative time period, the CAM boot is worn nightly to maintain ankle dorsiflexion. Beginning at 4 to 6 weeks postoperatively, focused plantar flexion muscle strength training can occur.[8,24,34]

OUTCOMES

There has been growing interest in performing surgical gastrocnemius lengthening to treat secondary metatarsalgia. Much of this interest stems from successful clinical outcomes when using the soft tissue lengthening procedures to address similar pathologies arising from forefoot overload. Mueller and colleagues[35] demonstrated

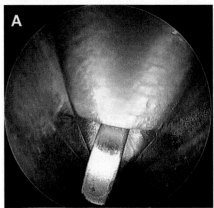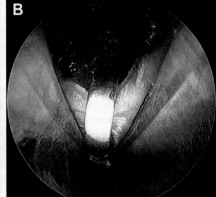

Fig. 6. Endoscopic gastrocnemius release: (*A*) Endoscopic image when the cannula is inserted deep to the crural fascia. (*B*) A retrograde knife is used to release the gastrocnemius tendon from the midline laterally.

improved healing and lower recurrence rates in patients with diabetic or neuropathic plantar ulcers treated with Achilles tendon lengthening as compared with their non-lengthened counterparts. Laborde[36] reported similar findings in diabetic patients who underwent gastrocnemius recession. Maskill and colleagues[8] performed surgical gastrocnemius lengthening for isolated foot pain in 29 patients with isolated gastrocnemius tightness and found that after an average of 19.5 months of follow-up, the average pain score improvement was from 8 to 2 on a scale of 10. Ninety-three percent of patients were satisfied with their results.[37] Surgical gastrocnemius lengthening in patients with recalcitrant foot pain experienced increased passive ankle dorsiflexion range of motion (average of 14°–18°), improved function with daily activities, and maintained plantar flexion strength.[8,30,38,39]

Morales-Muñoz and colleagues[13] studied the effectiveness of proximal gastrocnemius release in treating mechanical metatarsalgia and found a reduction in visual analog scale (VAS) pain scores and improvement in the American Orthopedic Foot and Ankle Society scores and average ankle dorsiflexion at 6 months postoperatively in their cohort of 52 patients (78 feet). Thirty-six (69.2%) patients reported satisfaction with the outcome of their surgery, and no patients reported worsening of their symptoms after surgery.[13] Forty-nine of 52 patients returned to active work duty without restriction by 1 month postoperatively.[13]

The outcomes on preserved plantar flexion strength following isolated gastrocnemius recession remain sparse. Sammarco and colleagues[40] found that, compared with the contralateral extremity, plantar flexion peak torque in the operative extremity increased to 82% of the nonoperative limb at 18 months postoperatively; however, the patients in this cohort underwent lengthening of both the gastrocnemius and soleus. In case-control series of 7 subjects who underwent isolated gastrocnemius recession, Chimera and colleagues[39] found that, although subjects had deficits in isometric and isokinetic plantar flexion strength preoperatively when compared with healthy control subjects, their isometric plantar flexion strength did not decrease postoperatively; however, their isokinetic plantar flexion strength significantly ($P = .018$) increased at 3 months postoperatively but still remained lower than that of healthy controls. This improvement in isokinetic strength is thought to be related to the plantar flexor muscles operating in a more favorable portion of the length tension curve.[39] Interestingly, these patients' self-reported level of function for activities of daily living and global rating of function increased by 35% and 45%, respectively, and approached the lower limit of scores in healthy control subjects.[39]

Although their reports may not be generalizable to patients with metatarsalgia, Nawoczenski and colleagues[15] reported significant pain reduction but with decreases in ankle plantar flexion strength in patients treated with a Strayer gastrocnemius recession for Achilles tendinopathy as compared with controls. The study groups noted no significant difference in ankle plantarflexion power between involved and uninvolved limbs of the gastrocnemius recession group during lower levels of activity, such as during walking and standard-step ascent; however, statistically significant plantar flexion differences were noted when patients were asked to negotiate steps of greater height.[15] Molund and Lapinskas[41] found different outcomes, however, regarding postoperative ankle plantar flexion strength. They studied 34 patients, representing 39 operated legs, who underwent Strayer gastrocnemius recession (35 open, 4 endoscopic) for chronic Achilles tendinopathy. Postoperatively, 10 patients underwent functional testing, which included vertical jump-countermovement jump, hopping, drop countermovement jump, concentric toe raise, eccentric concentric toe raise, and toe raise endurance.[41] In tested patients, they found no difference in gastrocsoleus complex function between operated and nonoperated legs; however, they do concede that their sample size was underpowered to detect statistically significant differences.[41]

Gastrocnemius lengthening performed endoscopically seems to be an effective alternative to open surgical technique. Phisitkul and colleagues[21] performed endoscopic gastrocnemius recession in 320 consecutive patients, 30 of which underwent the procedure for secondary metatarsalgia causing forefoot overloading. VAS pain scores decreased from a preoperative average of 7.0 to 4.2 postoperatively.[34] The 36-Item Short Form Survey and Foot Forum Index scores improved at a minimum of a 1-year follow-up.[21,34] Ankle dorsiflexion values improved from $-0.4°$ to $13.4°$ immediately postoperatively.[34] At the final follow-up, patients averaged $10.5°$ of ankle dorsiflexion.[34] The investigators reported that patients presenting with metatarsalgia and forefoot overloading symptoms seemed to directly benefit from gastrocnemius lengthening.[34]

Complications

Both open and endoscopic gastrocnemius recessions have been shown to have complication rates of 0% to 20%.[8,10,24,32] Complications of gastrocnemius recession include sural nerve injury, weakness, cosmesis, and muscle atrophy of the calf. Rush and colleagues[24] performed a retrospective review and examined 126 patients who underwent a Strayer procedure. They found that 6% of patients developed a postsurgical complication, including unsatisfactory scar cosmesis, wound dehiscence, infection, sural nerve injury, or complex regional pain syndrome. Saxena and colleagues[33] reported sural nerve injury in 11% of patients and unacceptable cosmesis due to scar adhesions in 11% of patients in 47 patients who underwent endoscopic gastrocnemius recession. Trevino and colleagues,[37] however, published a retrospective study of 28 patients who also underwent endoscopic gastrocnemius release; there was no incidence of sural nerve damage or subcutaneous dimpling at the scar at their final follow-up. Phisitkul and colleagues[21,34] reported complications after endoscopic gastrocnemius recession of ankle plantar flexion weakness and sural nerve dysesthesia reaching 3%; however, sural nerve complications were noted to have resolved by 1 year without further deficit. In a recent surgical strategies article describing endoscopic recession of the gastrocnemius tendon, the investigators deemed the procedure safe and effective to relieve pain due to isolated gastrocnemius contracture.[34]

SUMMARY

Surgical gastrocnemius lengthening to address secondary metatarsalgia seems to be safe and effective in patients who have failed nonoperative treatment modalities. Reducing weight-bearing plantar pressure, restoring foot biomechanics, and alleviation of forefoot pain are the goals of surgery. A Silfverskiold test must be performed preoperatively to determine if isolated gastrocnemius recession or Achilles tendon lengthening is indicated. Both open or minimally invasive endoscopic techniques may be used to release the gastrocnemius soft tissue structures. Regardless of technique, care must be taken to prevent injury to the sural nerve. Surgeons should select the operative technique that allows them to consistently perform a safe and effective surgery.

REFERENCES

1. Besse J. Metatarsalgia. Orthop Traumatol Surg Res 2017;103(1S):S29–39.
2. Espinosa N, Brodsky J, Maceira E. Metatarsalgia. J Am Acad Orthop Surg 2010; 18(8):474–85.

3. Espinosa N, Maceira E, Myerson M. Current concept review. Metatarsalgia. Foot Ankle Int 2008;29:871–9.
4. Scranton P. Metatarsalgia: a clinical review of diagnosis and management. Foot Ankle 1981;1(4):229–34.
5. Aronow MS, Diaz-Doran V, Sullivan RJ, et al. The effect of triceps surae contracture force on plantar foot pressure distribution. Foot Ankle Int 2006;27:43–52.
6. Ledoux WR, Shofer JB, Ahroni JH, et al. Biomechanical differences among pes cavus, neutrally aligned, and pes planus feet in subjects with diabetes. Foot Ankle Int 2003;24:845–50.
7. Downey M, Banks A. Gastrocnemius recession in the treatment of nonspastic ankle equinus: a retrospective study. J Am Podiatr Med Assoc 1989;79:159–74.
8. Maskill J, Bohay D, Anderson J. Gastrocnemius recession to treat isolated foot pain. Foot Ankle Int 2010;31(1):19–23.
9. DiGiovanni C, Kuo R, Tejwani N, et al. Isolated gastrocnemius tightness. J Bone Joint Surg Am 2002;84-A(6):962–70.
10. Hill R. Ankle equinus: prevalence and linkage to common foot pathology. J Am Podiatr Med Assoc 1995;85(6):295–300.
11. Cazeau C, Stiglitz Y. Effects of gastrocnemius tightness on forefoot of during gait. Foot Ankle Clin 2014;19(4):649–57.
12. Jastifer J, Marston J. Gastrocnemius contracture in patients with and without foot pathology. Foot Ankle Int 2016;37(11):1165–70.
13. Morales-Muñoz P, De Los Santos Real R, Sanz P, et al. Proximal gastrocnemius release in the treatment of mechanical metatarsalgia. Foot Ankle Int 2016;37(7): 782–9.
14. Silfverskiold N. Reduction of the uncrossed two joints muscles of the leg to one joint muscles in spastic conditions. Acta Chir Scand 1924;56:315–28.
15. Nawoczenski D, Diliberto F, Cantor M, et al. Ankle power and endurance outcomes following isolated gastrocnemius recession for Achilles tendinopathy. Foot Ankle Int 2016;37(7):766–75.
16. Gajdosik R, Allred J, Gabbert H, et al. A stretching program increases the dynamic passive length and passive resistive properties of the calf muscle-tendon unit of unconditioned younger women. Eur J Appl Physiol 2007;99: 449–54.
17. Dockery G. Evaluation and treatment of metatarsalgia and keratotic disorders. In: Myerson M, editor. Foot and ankle disorders. Philadelphia: Saunders; 2000. p. 359–77.
18. Harvey L, Herbert R, Crosbie J. Does stretching induce lasting increases in joint ROM? A systematic review. Physiother Res Int 2002;7(1):1–13.
19. Radford J, Burns J, Buchbinder R, et al. Does stretching increase ankle dorsiflexion range of motion? A systematic review. Br J Sports Med 2006;40(10):870–5 [discussion: 875].
20. Ivanic G, Trnka H, Homann N. Post-traumatic metatarsalgia: early results of treatment with a new insole. Unfallchirurg 2000;103:507–10 [German].
21. Phisitkul P, Barg A, Amendola A. Endoscopic recession of the gastrocnemius tendon. Foot Ankle Int 2017;38(4):457–64.
22. Hodge M, Bach T, Carter G. Novel Award first prize paper: orthotic management of plantar pressure and pain in rheumatoid arthritis. Clin Biomech (Bristol, Avon) 1999;14:567–75.
23. Kang J, Chen S, Hsi W. Correlations between subjective treatment responses and plantar pressure parameters of metatarsal pad treatment in metatarsalgia patients: a prospective study. BMC Musculoskelet Disord 2006;5:95.

24. Rush S, Ford L, Hamilton G. Morbidity associated with high gastrocnemius recession: retrospective review of 126 cases. J Foot Ankle Surg 2006;45(3):156–60.
25. Pinney S, Sangeorzan B, Hansen S. Surgical anatomy of the gastrocnemius recession (Strayer procedure). Foot Ankle Int 2004;25(4):247–50.
26. Vulpius OS, Stoffel A. Tenotomie der end schnen der mm: Gastrocnemius et soleus mittels rutschenlassens nach vulpius. In: Enke F, editor. Orthopadische Operationslehre. Germany: Stuttgart; 1913. p. 29–31.
27. Strayer L. Recession of the gastrocnemius: an operation to relieve spastic contracture of the calf muscles. J Bone Joint Surg Am 1950;32-A(3):671–6.
28. Baumann JU. Ventrale aponeurotische Verliingerung des Musculus gastrocnemius. Oper Orthop Traumatol 1989;1(4):254–8.
29. Barske H, DiGiovanni B. Current concept review: isolated gastrocnemius contracture and gastrocnemius recession. Foot Ankle Int 2012;33(10):915–21.
30. Herzenberg J, Lamm B, Corwin C, et al. Isolated recession of the gastrocnemius muscle: the Baumann procedure. Foot Ankle Int 2007;28(11):1154–9.
31. Abdulmassih S, Phisitkul P, Femino J, et al. Triceps surae contracture: implications for foot and ankle surgery. J Am Acad Orthop Surg 2013;21:398–407.
32. Tashjian R, Appel A, Banerjee R, et al. Endoscopic gastrocnemius recession: evaluation in a cadaver model. Foot Ankle Int 2003;24(8):607–13.
33. Saxena A, Gollwitzer H, Widtfeldt A, et al. Endoscopic gastrocnemius recession as therapy for gastrocnemius equines. Z Orthop Unfall 2007;145(4):499–504 [German].
34. Phisitkul P, Rungprai C, Femino J, et al. Endoscopic gastrocnemius recession for the treatment of isolated gastrocnemius contracture. Foot Ankle Int 2014;35(8):747–56.
35. Mueller MJ, Sinacore DR, Hastings MK, et al. Effect of Achilles tendon lengthening on neuropathic plantar ulcers: a randomized clinical trial. J Bone Joint Surg Am 2003;85(8):1436–45.
36. Laborde J. Neuropathic plantar forefoot ulcers treated with tendon lengthenings. Foot Ankle Int 2008;29(4):378–84.
37. Trevino S, Gibbs M, Panchbhavi V. Evaluation of results of endoscopic gastrocnemius recession. Foot Ankle Int 2005;26(5):359–64.
38. Pinney S, Hansen S, Sangeorzan B. The effect on ankle dorsiflexion of gastrocnemius recession. Foot Ankle Int 2002;23:26–9.
39. Chimera N, Castro M, Manal K. Function and strength following gastrocnemius recession for isolated gastrocnemius contracture. Foot Ankle Int 2010;31(5):377–84.
40. Sammarco G, Bagwe M, Sammarco V, et al. The effects of unilateral gastrosoleus recession. Foot Ankle Int 2006;27(7):508–11.
41. Molund M, Lapinskas S. Clinical and functional outcomes of gastrocnemius recession for chronic Achilles tendinopathy. Foot Ankle Int 2016;37(10):1091–7.

Treatment of Flexible Lesser Toe Deformities

Solenne Frey-Ollivier, MD[a],*, Fernanda Catena, MD[b],
Marianne Hélix-Giordanino, MD[a], Barbara Piclet-Legré, MD[a]

KEYWORDS

- Forefoot • Lesser toe • Claw toe • Hammer toe • Percutaneous

KEY POINTS

- The clinical descriptions of hammer toes, claw toes, and mallet toes are poor and inconsistent.
- Classification of lesser toe deformities must be done using both clinical and radiological evaluation.
- First-line treatment of flexible toe deformities should be based on a combination of special orthoses, taping, or strapping to improve toe alignment.
- Percutaneous tenotomies and/or osteotomies are mainly appropriate according to morphologic criteria (à la carte) but also according to etiologic and reducibility criteria.

INTRODUCTION

Lesser toe deformities are among the most common complaints presented to foot and ankle specialists.[1,2] However, there is great variety within this clinical entity. For every specific type of deformity, there could be a combination of soft tissues and bony procedures, chosen à la carte by the surgeon, according to the surgeon's preferences.

Understanding local anatomy and pathophysiology is essential to address these deformities correctly.[1–3] The deformities could be part of a rheumatologic syndrome (such as rheumatoid arthritis), neurologic involvement (such as cerebral palsy or Charcot-Marie-Tooth), or most commonly are a consequence of mechanical overload. They also can appear as isolated entities or be associated with other deformities of the hallux, midfoot, or hindfoot.

Conflicts of Interest: The authors have nothing to disclose.
[a] Centre du Pied, 68, rue du Commandant Rolland, Marseille 13008, France; [b] Orthopaedics and Sports Medecine Department, Hospital Nove de Julho, Sao Paulo, France
* Corresponding author.
E-mail address: solennefrey@gmail.com

When there is no neurologic involvement, most claw toe deformities usually follow a known sequence: the hyperextension at the metatarsophalangeal (MTP) joint, (mostly caused by a local overload) leads to a change of center of rotation, which generates a muscular imbalance within the joints between intrinsic and extrinsic muscles[2,4,5] (**Fig. 1**). This muscular imbalance leads to MTP hyperextension associated with flexion of proximal and/or distal interphalangeal (DIP) joints as extrinsic muscles overpower the intrinsic muscles.

This movement can be accompanied by lateral or medial deviation as the deformities progress, potentially caused by capsular attenuation. Chronic deformities tend to become rigid, and footwear may worsen clinical smptoms.[1,4]

CLASSIFICATION

The definitions of hammer toe, claw toe, and mallet toe have been, and continue to be, the most confusing area of pathology for those involved with foot and ankle care.[6]

The word claw is used in most countries. The usual definition of claw is a pointed and curved element at the end of the legs or fingers of some mammals (lion, cat, tiger), birds of prey (hawks, falcons), and some reptiles; it is also often used in reference to invertebrates (eg, scorpions, clamps crabs, and lobsters).

Between hammer toes, claw toes, and mallet toes, the descriptions of the deformities are poor and discordant.[1,7,8] The clinical, radiographic, and morphologic criteria are important to analyze to determine the correct surgical procedure for each patient. For improved surgical planning, the authors propose a new international classification that is currently being validated within the French Association of Foot and Ankle surgeons (AFCP) (**Table 1**).

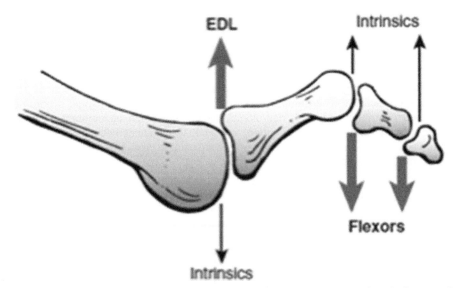

Fig. 1. The muscular unbalance leads to MTP hyperextension associated with flexion of proximal and/or distal interphalangeal joints, as extrinsic muscles (extensor digitorum longus [EDL], flexor digitorum brevis [FDB], and flexor digitorum longus [FDL]) dominate the intrinsic ones.

Table 1			
French Association of Foot and Ankle Surgeons classification for toe deformities			
Localization (Proximal to Distal)	**Deformation**	**Reducibility**	**Cause**
MP = meta-tarsophalangeal joint	f = flexion	f = flexible	rh = rheumatic
PIP = proximal interphalangeal	e = extension	sr = semirigid	pt = posttraumatic
DIP = distal interphalangeal	l = lateral deviation	r = rigid	nr = neurologic
	m = medial deviation		ic = iatrogenic

The description starts from proximal to distal: MP then PIP then DIP; and the number of the toe concerned must be added at the beginning of the description.

Morphologic Criteria

Metacarpophalangeal deformities

- MP: metacarpophalangeal joint in extension (the authors do use the letter e because this is the most frequent distortion)
- MP+: MP in extension with subluxation or dislocation
- MPl: MP in lateral subluxation
- MPm: MP in medial subluxation

Extension MP is rarely isolated (eg, 2MP; **Figs. 2** and **3**) and is usually associated with the proximal interphalangeal (PIP) (eg, 2MP PIP; **Fig. 4**).

- Lateral or medial MP subluxation without PIP (eg, 23MPl, **Fig. 5**; 2MPm, **Fig. 6**).
- Extension MP with subluxation or luxation (MP+) is usually clinically evident and confirmed with radiographs (**Fig. 7**).
- 2MP PIP (**Fig. 8**) may become 2MP+ PIP if the radiograph shows an MP subluxation (see **Fig. 8**; **Fig. 9**).

Proximal interphalangeal metacarpophalangeal deformities

- PIP: PIP in flexion (the authors do not use the letter f because this is the most frequent distortion)
- PIPe: PIP in extension (rare)
- PIPl: PIP in lateral subluxation
- PIPm: PIP in medial subluxation

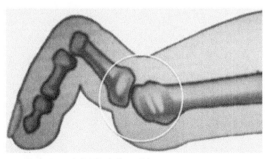

Fig. 2. The metacarpophalangeal (MP) deformities.

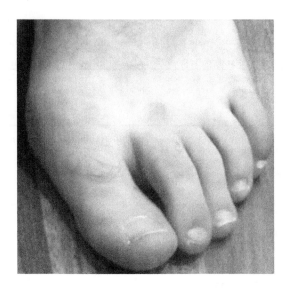

Fig. 3. 2MP.

PIP flexion deformities can be isolated (eg, 234PIP; **Fig. 10**) but are usually associated with MP deformities:

- In extension: 2MP PIP (see **Fig. 8**)
- With MP subluxation/luxation: 2MP+ PIP (see **Fig. 7**)
- With lateral deviation: 3MPl PIP (**Fig. 11**)
- With medial deviation: 23MPm PIP (**Fig. 12**)

In scientific publications, PIP deformity is often called hammer toe (eg, 234PIP; see **Fig. 10**), whereas claw toe is an MP PIP DIP deformity (eg, 2MP PIP DIP; **Fig. 13**). Mallet toe corresponds with a DIP deformity (eg, 2DIP; **Fig. 14**).[6]

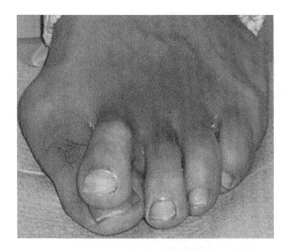

Fig. 4. 2MP PIP.

Distal interphalangeal deformities
• DIP: DIP in flexion (the authors do not use the letter f because this is the most frequent displacement)
• DIPe: DIP in extension (rare)
• DIPl: DIP in lateral subluxation
• DIPm: DIP in medial subluxation

Deformities may exist with 1, 2, or 3 levels of classification: examples include 2DIP (**Fig. 15**), 3DIPl (**Fig. 16**), 2PIP DIP (**Fig. 17**), 2MP PIP DIP, and MP+ PIP DIP (**Fig. 18**).

Optional Criteria

The reducibility criteria (flexible [f], semirigid [sr], rigid [r]) can be added after the morphologic criteria. Examples include 3PIP DIPsr and 3PIPr.

The etiologic criteria (rheumatic [rh], posttraumatic [pt], neurologic [nr], iatrogenic [ic]) can best be added before the morphologic criteria. Examples include 3 rh PIPr DIPsr, 3 pt PIPf, 2 ic MPm 2 nr PIP DIP.

TREATMENTS
Conservative Treatment

The main goal is to relieve local pain and improve the patient's quality of life. Nonoperative treatments should always be proposed as the first line of treatment.

- Patients with lesser toe deformities are encouraged to wear shoes with wide toe boxes to better accommodate and alleviate impingement of the digits.
- Special orthoses or insoles may also promote pain relief and gait improvement.
- Taping or strapping of the affected toes may improve alignment if they are flexible.

An elastic adhesive bandage helps to orient or reduce mobility. Introduced in 1970 by a Japanese chiropractor, Kenso Kase, these allow different actions according to the direction and elasticity of the bandage layers (**Fig. 19**).[9]

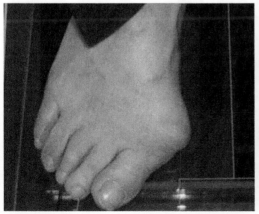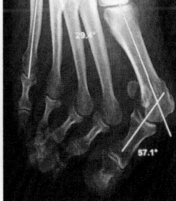

Fig. 5. 23MPl.

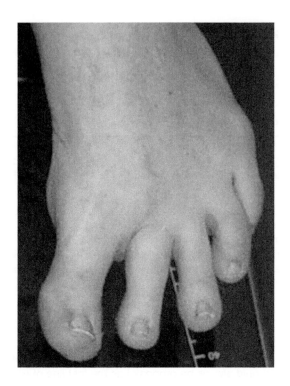

Fig. 6. 2MPm.

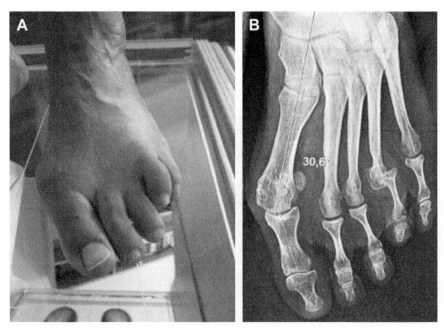

Fig. 7. (*A*) 4MP+ (*B*) PIP.

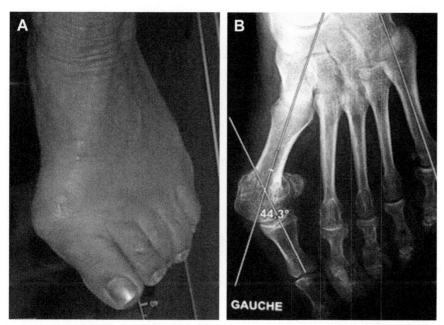

Fig. 8. (*A*) A patient with a classic clinical 2MP PIP but radiograph analysis (*B*) of the same patient shows an MP subluxation thus changing the classification from 2MP PIP to MP+ PIP.

- Rehabilitation can stop the aggravation of a flexible deformity. This approach is the Strain-Counterstrain technique developed by Jones and colleagues[10] of the American Academy of Osteopathy and introduced to surgeons by Dr. Michel Maestro. It consists of passive positioning that places the deformed toe in a position of maximum comfort (typically MP flexion), alleviating pain by reducing and stopping the inappropriate activity of the proprioceptor that maintains somatic dysfunction. By passively reproducing the initial tension position, the patient moves the joint into a more comfortable position that shortens the muscle involved as much as possible. Holding for 90 seconds allows the muscle spindle to slow down its associated discharge frequency. The return to the neutral position in a slow and deliberate manner avoids reexciting the previously spastic muscle fibers.[10] For a proximal deformity, the patient maintains the first 90 seconds by first performing slight traction along the longitudinal axis.

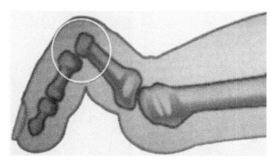

Fig. 9. The PIP deformities.

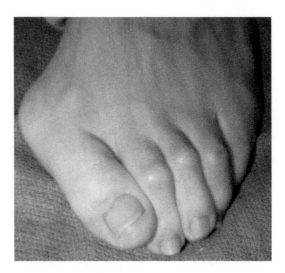

Fig. 10. 234PIP.

Surgical Treatment

When a surgical decision is made the patient's comorbidities must be considered, because postoperative complications are directly related to vascular or neurologic impairment. Careful physical examination is necessary to differentiate various deformities and understand their pathogenesis. For example, hallux deviation associated with lesser toe deformities must be corrected to obtain favorable outcomes even if it is not the main complaint.

The procedures may be used in various combinations to achieve a good correction. Both open and percutaneous surgical techniques are described, and can be

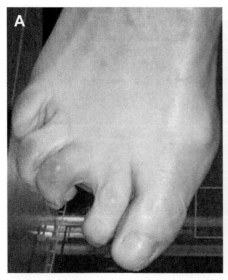
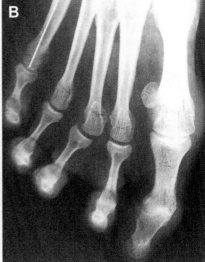

Fig. 11. (A, B) 3MPl PIP and other deformities (2MPmPIPDIP, 4MPlPIPDIP, 5PIPDIP).

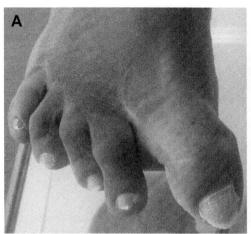
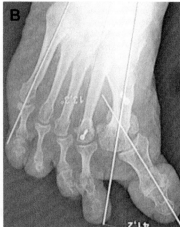

Fig. 12. (*A, B*) 23 MPm PIP.

subdivided into either soft tissue or bony procedures. However, all techniques share the same goal: realigning the toe in the least invasive manner possible, so the optimal combination is patient specific and unique for every deformity. If the MTP joint is dislocated, a metatarsal osteotomy will probably be needed to allow appropriate correction of the proximal phalanx position. Extension of the MTP joint might be corrected

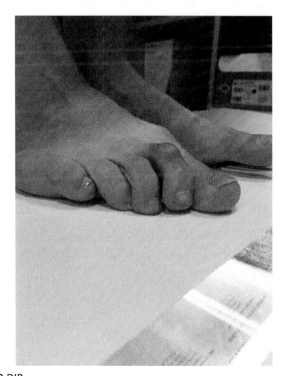

Fig. 13. 2MP PIP DIP.

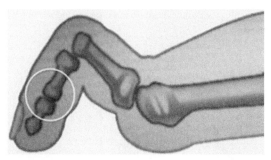

Fig. 14. The DIP deformities.

with tendon release or tendon transfer, or even adding proximal phalanx osteotomy. PIP joint flexion can be realigned using procedures ranging from plantar capsular release to resectional arthroplasties. Surgeons should master different techniques and plan corrections according to their experience.

Open surgery

Soft tissue procedures include tendon and capsular release, tendon transfer, and plantar plate repair. Most of the surgeries involve extensor tendon lengthening plus capsular release at the MTP joint and flexor tendon lengthening plus plantar capsular release at the PIP joint.

Tendon transfers are usually intended to stabilize the MTP joint by rebalancing the extrinsic and intrinsic forces.[11-15] This transfer also functions to correct the proximal

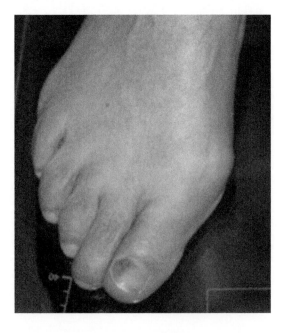

Fig. 15. 2DIP.

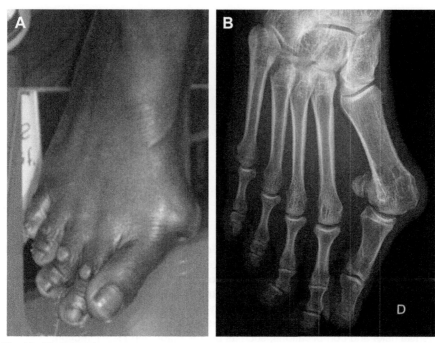

Fig. 16. (*A, B*) 3DIPI.

phalanx position and, consequently, the center of rotation of the MTP joint. Tendon transfers are described in more detail in Caio Nery and Daniel Baumfeld's article, "Lesser Metatarsophalangeal Joint Instability: Treatment with Tendon Transfers," in this issue.

Bony procedures include phalangeal osteotomies, metatarsal osteotomies (please see David Redfern's article, "Treatment of Metatarsalgia with Distal Osteotomies"; and Emily C. Vafek and Simon Lee's article, "Treatment of Metatarsalgia with Proximal Osteotomies," in this issue), and interphalangeal resection arthroplasties

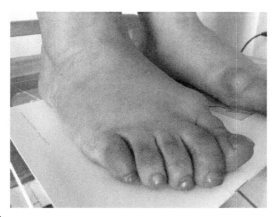

Fig. 17. 2 PIP DIP.

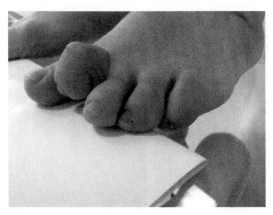

Fig. 18. MP + PIP DIP.

(please see Jesse F. Doty and Jason A. Fogleman's article, "Treatment of Rigid Hammer toe Deformity: Permanent vs. Removable Implant Selection," in this issue).

Proximal phalanx osteotomy is intended to shorten the toe and thus minimize the deforming forces of the surrounding soft tissues. The technique is described by Ceccarini and colleagues[16] with good short-term and long-term outcomes.

Most open surgeries include temporary Kirschner-wire fixation with the associated potential risks and complications, such as pin migration and local infection.[17,18]

Recent studies have shown the importance of plantar plate attenuation or rupture on lesser toe deformity pathogenesis. The disruption of the plantar plate may be addressed depending on lesion severity.[19–21] MTP arthroscopy may be used as a diagnostic method as well as a surgical approach for plantar plate shrinkage.[21] The open approach can be performed dorsally or plantarly.[2,20,22,23] The goals of the surgery are first to repair the plantar structures to correct toe alignment and optimize muscular balance. This technique is often performed in combination with a Weil osteotomy in order to better access the plantar plate, increase joint space, and reduce the MTP joint.[19]

Percutaneous surgery
Soft tissues procedures Isolated tenotomy of the extensor digitorum longus (FDB) **(Fig. 20)**: with the toe positioned in strict plantar flexion during the whole procedure to avoid injury of the plantar collateral nerve, the incision is made proximal to the

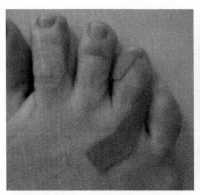
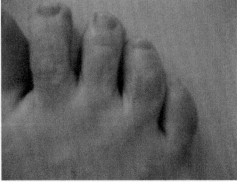

Fig. 19. K-taping for a 4PIP.

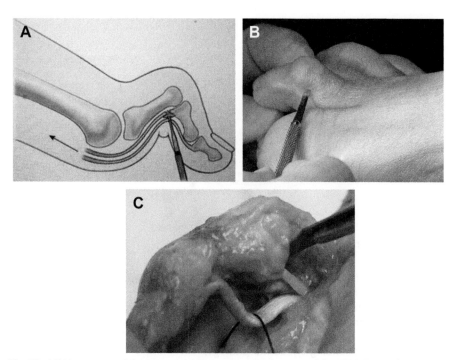

Fig. 20. (*A*) Tenotomy of the FDB and (*B*) plantar capsulotomy of the PIP joint with a Beaver; (*C*) lateral or medial incision, toe in plantar flexion.

PIP joint (see **Fig. 20**), lateral or medial depending of the surgeon's dominant hand. With the opposite hand, the surgeon palpates the tubercle of the distal epiphysis of P1.

The Beaver blade is then introduced directly plantar to the P1 neck, maintaining contact with the bone. Then, following the plantar surface of P1 distally to the plantar base of P2, the PIP plantar capsule and FDB are released through a rotational motion. A periosteal elevator is then introduced to check the complete section of the 2 limbs of the FDB, by careful palpation of the entire plantar surface of P2 diaphysis, including its lateral and medial edges. The complete release of the interphalangeal capsule (arthrolysis) is a prerequisite for reaching P2 diaphysis and the distal insertion of the FDB's 2 limbs in relation to the capsule (see **Fig. 20**). The released toe is then brought into dorsiflexion by a passive maneuver in order to check the reduction of the PIP joint.

The isolated FDB tenotomy can also be performed by the plantar approach at the base of P1 where the FDB is on the surface, but there is a higher risk of not being selective. In addition, plantar arthrolysis of the PIP joint cannot be performed at this level, which is an important step to correct the deformity.

Isolated tenotomy of the flexor digitorum longus (FDL) (**Fig. 21**): performed by a distal plantar incision at the level of the distal interphalangeal joint or an incision comparable with that used for the FDB, but more distal. This procedure can be performed laterally or medially depending on the operated foot and the dominant hand of the surgeon, in order to reach the plantar surface of the base of P3.

Complete tenotomy (FDL and FDB): as shown by de Prado and colleagues,[24] the tenotomy is performed by a plantar incision at the base of the toe at the level of P1 (**Fig. 22**), which allows for sectioning of both the FDL and FDB, followed by dorsiflexion maneuver of the toe.

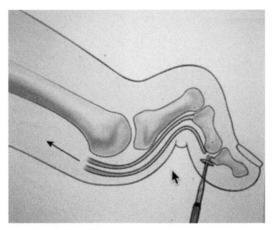

Fig. 21. Isolated tenotomy on the FDL.

The tenotomy of the extensors is performed in the zone where the 2 tendons (longus and brevis) are found (**Fig. 23**), at the level of the fibroaponeurotic strap over the MTP joint, to avoid a proximal retraction of the tendons and a falling or drop toe. A plantar flexion force is simultaneously performed to determine the optimal result of the procedure: criteria of success are first tactile (disappearance of the tendinous tension) and then visual, depending on toe morphology.

Dorsal capsule arthrolysis of the MTP joint is the logical deep extension of the extensor tenotomy, but sometimes the extensors are laterally offset. Therefore, longitudinal traction or reduction of the toe allows for entry of the Beaver blade into the MTP joint in certain cases of dislocated toes.

Osteotomies
Proximal phalanx The osteotomy of the proximal phalanx (P1) is performed by a plantar approach at the base of the toe, in the proximal metaphysis of P1 (**Fig. 24**). To avoid the flexor tendons, the toe is held in dorsiflexion and the Beaver blade is inserted longitudinally via a medial or lateral incision, depending on the side being operated on and the surgeon's dominant hand.

A rasp is then introduced in order to prepare the working area, in which a suitable burr begins the osteotomy at the edge of the phalanx, remaining in contact with the

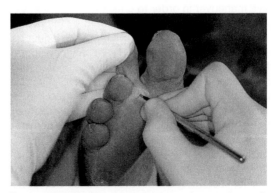

Fig. 22. Complete flexor tenotomy by a percutaneous plantar approach.

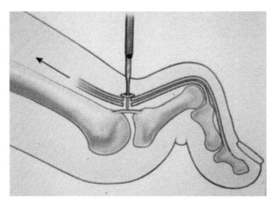

Fig. 23. Extensor tenotomy: dorsal incision at the MTP joint.

bone during the entire procedure. The osteotomy is best located at the proximal meta-physeal part of P1 to optimize the consolidation time.

- Monocortical osteotomy is sufficient to correct moderate deformities and allows correction of a lateral or medial MP deformity (**Fig. 25**).
- Bicortical osteotomy is most often used because it is an easier technique but also in order to obtain the shortening effect necessary for correction in more severe deformations or an excessively long toe (**Fig. 26**).

Middle phalanx The osteotomy of the middle phalanx (P2) is performed by a lateral or medial approach, depending on the operated foot and the desired deformity correction. It is mid-diaphyseal to avoid the articular surfaces (**Fig. 27**).

- Monocortical osteotomy allows dorsiflexion or correction of lateral or medial deformity of the DIP. This osteotomy also allows the reduction of a lateral or medial subluxation of the DIP if associated with release of the DIP joint (see **Fig. 16**; **Fig. 28**).
- Bicortical osteotomy: allows the shortening of a long middle phalanx.

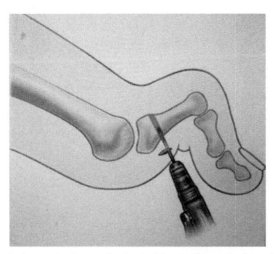

Fig. 24. Proximal phalanx osteotomy: plantar incision in the metaphyseal area.

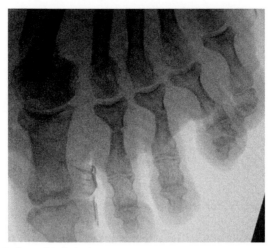

Fig. 25. Monocortical proximal phalanx osteotomy.

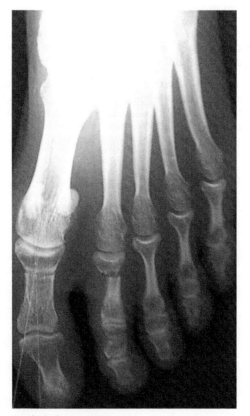

Fig. 26. Bicortical proximal phalanx osteotomy.

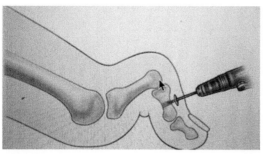

Fig. 27. Medial phalanx osteotomy: dorsomedial or dorsolateral incision.

Condylectomy Performing a condylectomy is uncommonly required in flexible deformities. The condylectomy can be performed by a lateral approach more distal than those used for P2 osteotomy. The incision is located at the level of the dorsal aspect of the P2 neck. From this point it is possible to remove the protruding dorsal part of the P1 head, as well as a portion of the P2 base. Bone debris is removed carefully, aided by palpation around the joint. However, inadequate removal of all bone debris is possible and can subsequently lead to discomfort in contact with the shoe. This condyloplasty is sometimes easier by a dorsal approach, distal to the P2 base with the toe flexed.

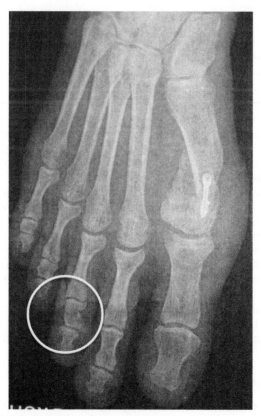

Fig. 28. Radiographs of a medial phalanx osteotomy.

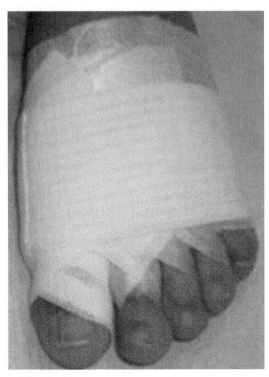

Fig. 29. Postoperative dressing.

Postoperative care The postoperative dressing is important to ensure success (**Fig. 29**), thus surgeons should perform it in the operating room. The dressing is replaced 1 week later by a trained nurse. The dressing is left for 3 weeks then replaced with an orthosis designed by a pedorthist in the presence of the surgeon (**Fig. 30**). Patients are instructed to keep their orthoses on day and night for 3 more weeks. Home active autorehabilitation begins according to physiotherapist instructions explained immediately after the surgery. After the second dressing (8 days), the authors teach patients (or their partners) to mobilize their operated toes twice a day. A physiotherapist can perform massage and rehabilitation after 21 days with precise instructions.

Postoperative shoe type depends of whether first ray surgery was performed in conjunction with the lesser toe surgery; typically, the authors allow weight bearing as tolerated in a stiff postoperative shoe. Radiographs are taken at 21 and 45 days; bone healing may be delayed. Depending on sport activities, a new radiograph is typically performed at 3 months, 6 months, or 1 year.

Collaboration between the surgeon, nurse, and pedorthist is necessary during the first 45 days for a good result. After this time period, the operated toe is sometimes held with strapping, an orthosis, and/or a night support in order to maintain a good position.

SURGICAL DECISION MAKING BASED ON DEFORMITY

Tenotomies and/or osteotomies are mainly appropriate according to morphologic criteria (à la carte) but also according to causal and reducibility criteria (**Fig. 31**).

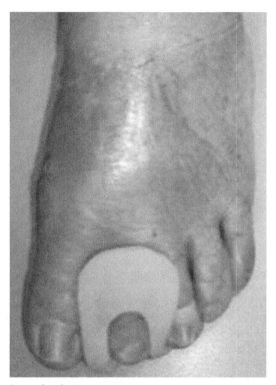

Fig. 30. Postoperative orthoplasty.

Morphologic Criteria

PIP are the most common deformities. Appropriate percutaneous procedures are selective FDB tenotomy in conjunction with plantar PIP release, which allows for correction of PIP flexion. P1 osteotomy may allow for a more durable correction.

An additional P2 osteotomy is useful when the correction is insufficient. Condyloplasty is an articular PIP procedure with few indications for use, especially in flexible deformities.

For MP PIP, additional extensors tenotomies are likely to be necessary.

For isolated MP(e) without PIP, extensor tenotomies are usually enough; once the tenotomy is performed, the authors determine whether an additional monocortical P1-lowering osteotomy is required.

For MP+ PIP, after tenotomies, a second step can be done to improve reduction of the deformity: MP release, metatarsal neck osteotomy, or open osteotomy. Surgeons determine which second step to perform based on the amount of MP dislocation.

Dorsal MP release can be unsafe if not justified. A partially dislocated toe may become dislocated after MP release. This procedure should be carefully considered, and the authors reserve it for MP dislocations. Some lateral or medial MP deformities may justify a selected MP release with a strict postoperative dressing, holding the MP joint in a plantar or neutral position. However, MP release is usually not necessary because MP reduction is obtained by P1 osteotomies, often associated with distal metatarsal osteotomies.

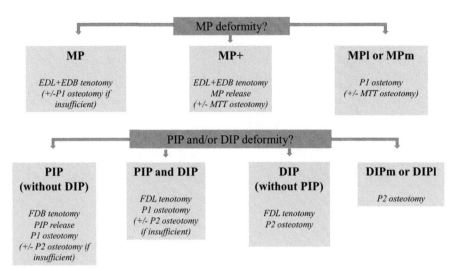

Fig. 31. Lasser toe deformity treatment algorithm.

DIP deformities are corrected with P2 osteotomy and/or selective FDL tenotomy.

Complex deformities (PIPDIP, MP+ PIP DIP) are typically approached with selected procedures; for example, for an MP PIP DIP, the authors recommend a total flexor tenotomy (FDB+ FDL)and P1 osteotomy plus or minus P2.

Flexibility Criteria

Very flexible deformities are usually corrected with a simple phalanx osteotomy (P1 or P2).

Causal Criteria

The cause can guide procedure choice; tenotomies are typically indicated for neurologic cases, whereas osteophytes present radiographically may change the decision to perform percutaneous surgery.

AUTHORS' EXPERIENCE

The authors have used percutaneous surgery for lesser toe deformities since 2004. In 2015, Frey and colleagues[25] published a series of 57 feet presenting with isolated second toe PIP deformity without metatarsalgia or DIP deformity treated with the technique discussed earlier. Mean age was 64.4 years and mean follow-up was 30.7 months. Procedures performed included selective FDB tenotomy, plantar PIP release, and P1 osteotomy. Extensor tenotomy was performed in 42% cases. Effective morphologic correction was obtained in 89.5% cases, with the same rate for global satisfaction. Active plantar flexion was preserved in 86% of cases and the authors noted only 12% of toes with postoperative stiffness (rigid PIP with no passive flexion) even though 74% of the toes were preoperatively semirigid or rigid. Two failures (3.5%) were revised with PIP fusion.

CONTRAINDICATIONS FOR PERCUTANEOUS TOE SURGERY

Open procedures may be preferred to correct articular deformities with proliferative osteoarthritis. Percutaneous surgery in these cases might lead to a higher risk of osseous debris disturbing shoe wearing despite meticulous debridement. Open procedures are likely also to be preferred in revision surgery. Fusion may be decided in cases of severe articular damage or articular malunion, as well as in neurologic diseases like Parkinson in order to neutralize contractures. Because the patient's compliance is mandatory to obtain optimal outcomes, the authors do not recommend this type of procedure for noncompliant patients and those unable to attend routine follow-up visits.

MIXED SURGERY CONCEPT

Percutaneous procedures for lesser toe deformities may be combined with other procedures, such as metatarsal osteotomies, bunion surgery, and gastrocnemius lengthening.

SUMMARY

The high variability of lesser toe deformities necessitates that surgeons develop an individualized, step-by-step approach to each patient. Deformity classification is mandatory for surgical preparation: in our daily practice, localization, type of deformity, reducibility, and cause must be detailed to determine operative decision making. Once classified, a specific combination of soft tissue and bony procedures can be chosen à la carte by the surgeon.

REFERENCES

1. Coughlin MJ, Saltzman CL, Mann RA. Mann's surgery of the foot and ankle E-book: expert consult - online. Elsevier Health Sciences; 2013.
2. Doty JF, Coughlin MJ, Weil L, et al. Etiology and management of lesser toe metatarsophalangeal joint instability. Foot Ankle Clin 2014;19(3):385–405.
3. Sarrafian SK, Topouzian LK. Anatomy and physiology of the extensor apparatus of the toes. J Bone Joint Surg Am 1969;51(4):669–79.
4. Wang B, Guss A, Chalayon O, et al. Deep transverse metatarsal ligament and static stability of lesser metatarsophalangeal joints: a cadaveric study. Foot Ankle Int 2015;36(5):573–8.
5. Nery C, Coughlin M, Baumfeld D, et al. How to classify plantar plate injuries: parameters from history and physical examination. Rev Bras Ortop 2015;50(6):720–8.
6. Malhotra K, Davda K, Singh D. The pathology and management of lesser toe deformities. EFORT Open Rev 2016;1(11):409–19.
7. Schuberth JM. Hammer toe syndrome. J Foot Ankle Surg 1999;38(2):166–78.
8. Pathologie du pied et de la cheville - Table des matières - EM consulte. Available at: http://www.em-consulte.com/livre/461208/table-des-matieres/pathologie-du-pied-et-de-la-cheville-. Accessed May 15, 2017.
9. Reuter BH. Taping the hammer toe. J Athl Train 1995;30(2):178–9.
10. Jones LH, Kusunose RS, Goering EK. Jones strain-counterstrain. Boise (ID): Jones Strain Counterstrain; 1995.
11. Veljkovic A, Lansang E, Lau J. Forefoot tendon transfers. Foot Ankle Clin 2014;19(1):123–37.
12. Hobizal KB, Wukich DK, Manway J. Extensor digitorum brevis transfer technique to correct multiplanar deformity of the lesser digits. Foot Ankle Spec 2016;9(3):252–7.

13. Butterworth M. Tendon transfers for management of digital and lesser metatarsophalangeal joint deformities. Clin Podiatr Med Surg 2016;33(1):71–84.
14. Myers SH, Schon LC. Forefoot tendon transfers. Foot Ankle Clin 2011;16(3): 471–88.
15. Trasposizione del flessore lungo dell'alluce (FLA) alla falange basale pro flessore breve - Chirurgia del Piede 2009;33(2):95–6-Minerva Medica - Riviste. Available at: http://www.minervamedica.it/it/riviste/chirurgia-piede/articolo.php?cod= R32Y2009N02A0095&acquista=1. Accessed May 15, 2017.
16. Ceccarini P, Ceccarini A, Rinonapoli G, et al. Correction of hammer toe deformity of lateral toes with subtraction osteotomy of the proximal phalanx neck. J Foot Ankle Surg 2015;54(4):601–6.
17. Kramer WC, Parman M, Marks RM. Hammertoe correction with K-wire fixation. Foot Ankle Int 2015;36(5):494–502.
18. Holinka J, Schuh R, Hofstaetter JG, et al. Temporary Kirschner wire transfixation versus strapping dressing after second MTP joint realignment surgery: a comparative study with ten-year follow-up. Foot Ankle Int 2013;34(7):984–9.
19. Nery C, Raduan FC, Catena F, et al. Plantar plate radiofrequency and Weil osteotomy for subtle metatarsophalangeal joint instability. J Orthop Surg 2015;10:180.
20. Nery C, Coughlin MJ, Baumfeld D, et al. Lesser metatarsophalangeal joint instability: prospective evaluation and repair of plantar plate and capsular insufficiency. Foot Ankle Int 2012;33(4):301–11.
21. Lui TH. Arthroscopic-assisted correction of claw toe or overriding toe deformity: plantar plate tenodesis. Arch Orthop Trauma Surg 2007;127(9):823–6.
22. Chalayon O, Chertman C, Guss AD, et al. Role of plantar plate and surgical reconstruction techniques on static stability of lesser metatarsophalangeal joints: a biomechanical study. Foot Ankle Int 2013;34(10):1436–42.
23. Flint WW, Macias DM, Jastifer JR, et al. Plantar plate repair for lesser metatarsophalangeal joint instability. Foot Ankle Int 2017;38(3):234–42.
24. de Prado M, Ripoll PL, Golanó P. Cirugía percutánea del pie: técnicas quirúrgicas, indicaciones, bases anatómicas. Masson; 2003. Available at: https:// dialnet.unirioja.es/servlet/libro?codigo=134516. Accessed May 2, 2017.
25. Frey S, Hélix-Giordanino M, Piclet-Legré B. Percutaneous correction of second toe proximal deformity: proximal interphalangeal release, flexor digitorum brevis tenotomy and proximal phalanx osteotomy. Orthop Traumatol Surg Res 2015; 101(6):753–8.

Treatment of Rigid Hammer-Toe Deformity

Permanent Versus Removable Implant Selection

Jesse F. Doty, MD*, Jason A. Fogleman, MD

KEYWORDS

- Hammer toe • Interphalangeal • Fusion • Implant • Rigid

KEY POINTS

- The type of surgical intervention is determined by the relative flexibility of the deformity and the presence or absence of associated metatarsophalangeal joint deformity or instability.
- Patients must have adequate vascularity to heal surgical sites before successfully addressing hammer-toe deformity.
- Fixed hammer-toe deformities can be successfully treated with proximal interphalangeal joint resection arthroplasty or fusion, with high patient satisfaction and low complication rates.
- Patient satisfaction does not depend on proximal interphalangeal joint bony fusion, as fibrous unions often remain asymptomatic; but malalignment is often poorly tolerated.
- Temporary Kirschner-wire fixation remains extremely popular for hammer-toe correction, but multiple permanent implants exist with high efficacy rates.

INTRODUCTION

A hammer toe is defined as either a rigid or flexible deformity of the lesser toes involving flexion of the proximal interphalangeal (PIP) joint. Anatomic or neuromuscular abnormalities lead to an imbalance in the intrinsic and extrinsic forces exerted on the toe. The intrinsic muscles of the foot (ie, lumbrical and interosseous musculature), through their tendinous orientation to the metatarsophalangeal (MTP), PIP, and distal interphalangeal (DIP) joint centers of rotation in the sagittal plane, act to flex the MTP joint and extend the PIP and DIP joints. The extensor digitorum longus (EDL) muscle via the extensor sling provides the primary MTP joint extension force. When

Disclosure Statement: Dr J.F. Doty is a paid consultant for Globus Medical Inc, Wright Medical Group, and Arthrex. Dr J.A. Fogleman has nothing to disclose.
Department of Orthopedic Surgery, Erlanger Health System, The University of Tennessee College of Medicine, 975 East Third Street, Hospital Box 260, Chattanooga, TN 37403, USA
* Corresponding author. 4986 Hamillville Court, Hixson, TN 37343.
E-mail address: jessd90@hotmail.com

Foot Ankle Clin N Am 23 (2018) 91–101
https://doi.org/10.1016/j.fcl.2017.09.007
1083-7515/18/© 2017 Elsevier Inc. All rights reserved.

the MTP joint is in an extended position, excursion of the EDL and the extensor sling is limited; thus, the EDL can only effectively function to extend the PIP and DIP joints when the MTP joint is in a neutral or a flexed position. The flexor digitorum longus (FDL) and flexor digitorum brevis muscles act as flexors of the DIP and PIP joints, respectively. An imbalance in these forces with respect to the hammer-toe deformity favors the stronger extrinsic muscles resulting in a PIP joint flexion deformity with possible MTP joint hyperextension[1] (**Fig. 1**).

Flexible hammer toes are passively correctable and may only be present with weight bearing. The distinction between the fixed and flexible deformity may help guide surgical intervention. Although flexible deformities may be amenable to correction through tenotomies, tendon transfers, resection arthroplasty, or fusions,[2] fixed deformities may only be amenable to resection arthroplasty or fusion to maintain successful correction of the underlying PIP joint flexion deformity.[3] The hammer toe can be further characterized as simple or complex depending on the presence of associated MTP joint hyperextension. The complex variant of the hammer-toe deformity causes some loss of clarity about the classic definitions of hammer-toe versus claw-toe deformities. Both entities are characterized by a PIP joint flexion deformity with associated MTP joint hyperextension deformity. However, although claw toes have simultaneous MTP joint hyperextension and DIP joint flexion deformities, hammer toes will exhibit either MTP joint hyperextension or DIP joint flexion but generally not both concurrently.[4] Furthermore, although both hammer-toe and claw-toe deformities can be associated with underlying neuromuscular disorders, inflammatory arthritides, and metabolic dysfunction, the claw toe is often more severe and more frequently involves multiple toes on bilateral feet.

PREOPERATIVE EVALUATION

Not all hammer-toe deformities are the same, and although hammer-toe correction can be straight forward, it is crucial to understand the nature of the deformity to achieve a successful outcome. The preoperative evaluation should involve not only the evaluation of the involved toe but a full history and examination of patients should also be performed to assess for pathology that could be contributing to the lesser toe deformity.

History should emphasize
- Medical comorbidities
- History of trauma, neuromuscular, and vascular disease
- Functional level

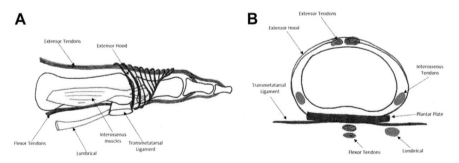

Fig. 1. Lesser-toe anatomy. (*A*) Lateral view. (*B*) Axial cut through metatarsal head. (*Courtesy of* Chase Kluemper MD, Department of Orthopedic Surgery, Erlanger Hospital, University of Tennessee, Chattanooga, TN.)

- Employment and recreational expectations
- Tobacco use
- Typical shoe wear
- Disease timing and symptom specifics
- Prior treatments to the foot

Physical examination should emphasize
- Neurologic examination (Is there underlying neuromuscular disease?)
- Vascular examination (Does adequate tissue perfusion exist to heal surgical wounds?)
- Ankle, hindfoot, midfoot examination (ie, pes cavus or pes planovalgus deformity)
- Forefoot evaluation
  - Inspection (gross deformity, callus or ulcer formation, surgical scars) (**Fig. 2**)
  - Palpation (Are there associated areas of tenderness?)
  - Hallux deformity
  - Flexible versus fixed deformity
  - MTP involvement
    - MTP deformity (ie, hyperextension, subluxation, dislocation, crossover toe)
    - MTP stability (drawer test)

Hammer toes can be associated with neuromuscular disorders, inflammatory arthritides, metabolic disorders, congenital abnormalities, and posttraumatic sequelae. Additional focused history will help determine if patients are surgical candidates or if patients might be better served with ongoing conservative management. A history of vascular disease, especially when combined with tobacco use, could place patients at particularly high risk for adverse outcomes when managed surgically. Prior surgery on the foot could drastically alter the approach to deformity correction.

The presence of associated hindfoot, midfoot, or forefoot deformities should be addressed at the time of hammer-toe correction or before hammer-toe correction to promote satisfactory correction and prevent recurrence of the deformity. Cavus foot deformity and hallux valgus are both commonly seen with hammer toes and can contribute to operative failure if not addressed concurrently. By definition, some degree of PIP joint flexion is present; but it is crucial to assess the MTP joint for associated hyperextension or instability. MTP joint instability may be present in the absence of transverse and sagittal plane deformity. The vertical drawer stress test is performed by stabilizing the metatarsal with one hand while placing a dorsal directed force on the

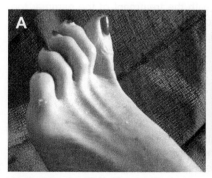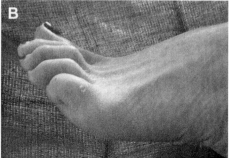

Fig. 2. Callus formation overlying the PIP joint in a hammer-toe deformity. (*A*) Dorsal view of left foot. (*B*) Lateral view of left foot.

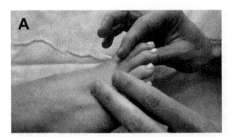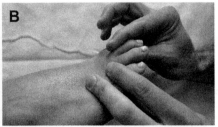

Fig. 3. MTP drawer test. (*A*) Grip the proximal phalanx between index and thumb and apply dorsally directed force on toe. (*B*) Subluxation of the MTP joint is assessed.

proximal phalanx of the toe (**Fig. 3**). Positive findings may include palpable instability or pain elicited by the maneuver. If present, MTP joint pathology is generally addressed before the PIP joint pathology. Flexible hammer-toe deformities can be managed with tenotomy or tendon transfer procedures, whereas fixed deformities often require PIP joint resection or fusion to correct the deformity.

Imaging should include anteroposterior, oblique, and lateral weight-bearing radiographs of the foot. If there is clinical suspicion of hindfoot malalignment, a weight-bearing hindfoot alignment radiograph can help further define the hindfoot position. Advanced imaging is rarely indicated for the workup of hammer toes in the absence of associated pathologic findings.

SURGICAL INDICATIONS

- Impending soft tissue compromise
- Failed nonoperative treatment with continued pain and deformity

PREOPERATIVE PLANNING

A flexible deformity can often be treated with a tenotomy or tendon transfer procedure. This procedure is described in greater detail in the article by Solenne Frey-Ollivier, Fernanda Catena, Marianne Hélix-Giordanino, et al, "Treatment of Flexible Lesser Toe Deformities," in this issue. A fixed hammer toe will not correct passively; therefore, tendon transfer alone will not correct the PIP joint flexion deformity. The standard for treatment of the fixed hammer toe is PIP joint resection arthroplasty or PIP joint fusion. An ipsilateral foot deformity, such as an associated cavus foot or hallux valgus, should be addressed before or concurrently with the treatment of the hammer toe. MTP joint deformity or instability should also be addressed concurrently with the hammer-toe correction. Treatment of MTP joint pathology may include

- Capsular release
- Extensor tendon lengthening
- Tendon transfer
- Weil osteotomy of the metatarsal
- Plantar plate repair

For further detail on addressing MTP joint pathology please see Caio Nery and Daniel Baumfeld's article, "Lesser Metatarsophalangeal Joint Instability: Treatment with Tendon Transfers"; and Raymond Y. Hsu and colleagues' article, "Lesser Metatarsophalangeal Joint Instability: Advancements in Plantar Plate Reconstruction", both in this issue.

SURGICAL TREATMENT

The authors' preferred technique for the primary treatment of fixed hammer-toe deformity (**Fig. 4**) is as follows:

1. Patients are placed in the supine position with a thigh or calf tourniquet. The procedure is performed under general anesthesia or regional block.
2. Preferably, a longitudinal incision is made over the dorsal surface of the PIP joint. However, an elliptical incision is also acceptable for excision of the dorsal callus that is often present.
3. The extensor hood and joint capsule are excised exposing the PIP joint.
4. The collateral ligaments are released off of the proximal phalanx, and the articular surface of the proximal phalanx is delivered.
5. Bone-cutting forceps are used to excise the distal articular surface of the proximal phalanx with a transverse cut across the metaphyseal region of the bone.
6. The articular surface at the base of the middle phalanx is removed with a small rongeur.
7. If the fusion surfaces cannot be opposed, a plantar capsulotomy and FDL tenotomy can be performed through the PIP joint.
8. A 0.062-in K-wire is introduced proximal to distal through the middle and distal phalanx and out of the tip of the toe. It is the authors' preference to use 0.062-in K-wires for all toes, although some surgeons suggest 0.045-in K-wires for smaller toes.
9. The PIP joint is reduced, and the K-wire is then advanced proximally across the PIP joint. The pin can be bent at the tip of the toe to prevent proximal migration.

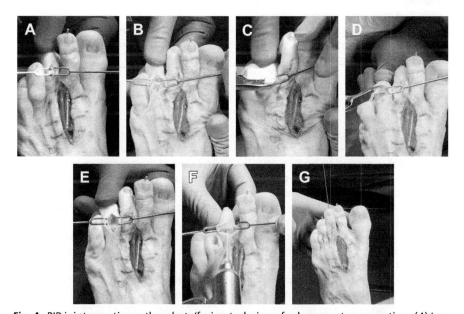

Fig. 4. PIP joint resection arthroplasty/fusion technique for hammer-toe correction. (*A*) Longitudinal incision overlying PIP joint. (*B*) Ellipse out extensor mechanism and joint capsule. (*C*) Expose distal articular surface of proximal phalanx and resect using bone cutting forceps. (*D*) Remove articular surface from middle phalanx using rongeur. (*E*) Joint prepared. (*F*) Introduce 0.045-in K-wire through middle phalanx and out of toe tip. (*G*) Reduce joint and pass K-wire in a retrograde fashion across PIP joint.

10. The incision is then closed with a nylon suture.
11. The tourniquet is released and the viability of toe perfusion is evaluated by color assessment. Toes that appear to remain pale in color are first manually manipulated and milked in attempt to restore color while maintaining surgical correction. The surgeon can release the tourniquet and any constrictive drapes while ensuring that there are no leg bumps or padding contributing to constricted popliteal flow. The leg is held over the side of the operating table, with the knee bent and the foot in a dependent position well below the heart, to incorporate gravitational forces in raising capillary pressure. The anesthesia team engages in allowing the systolic blood pressure to increase, which may be less than 100 mm Hg depending on the type of anesthetic used. It is the authors' experience that most sluggish toes generally improve at this point. Transdermal nitroglycerin may be applied to the toe to improve perfusion. Those patients with delayed capillary refill or delayed perfusion postsurgically are often admitted for observation with hourly vascular checks and heat-lamp application. In those rare scenarios, whereby the toe continues to be dysvascular, the decision must be discussed with patients and families of removing K-wires or passively manipulating the toe back into the presurgical anatomic position in an effort to restore flow and maintain viability. Some patients may choose to maintain surgical correction with an understanding of the possibility of necrosis and eventual amputation.

POSTOPERATIVE CARE

1. Soft dressing consisting of a non-adherent dressing, gauze, and tape is applied to the toe; a postoperative shoe or boot is used depending on the concurrent procedures that may have been performed.
2. Weight bearing through the heel is allowed if not precluded by other procedures.
3. A wound check and toe alignment is evaluated at 3 to 5 days postoperatively.
4. Stitches are removed at 2 to 3 weeks postoperatively
5. The K-wire is removed at 4 to 6 weeks postoperatively

OUTCOMES

Correction of the fixed hammer-toe deformity via PIP joint resection arthroplasty or arthrodesis is a highly effective procedure with patient satisfaction and pain resolution rates routinely reported to be 80% to 90%.[5,6] The goal of the procedure is to resolve the PIP joint flexion deformity by producing ankylosis of the joint in a neutral or slightly flexed position with minimal coronal plane deformity. Patient satisfaction does seem to correlate with coronal and sagittal plane alignment of the toe, but it may not depend on bony fusion of the joint.[5]

Coughlin and associates[5] reported on a series of 118 fixed hammer toes treated with PIP joint resection arthroplasty and K-wire stabilization. At an average 5-year follow-up, they reported an 81% radiographic fusion rate with fibrous union occurring in the remaining 19%. Radiographic alignment was noted by the clinician to be good in 79% of the toes, whereas patient-rated subjective alignment was acceptable in 86% of the toes. Pain relief was achieved in 92% of the patients, and 84% of the patients reported being satisfied with the overall outcome. Pain relief and patient satisfaction were similar in both patients with bony and fibrous unions.[5]

Ohm and associates[6] reported similar findings on a series of 25 patients treated with PIP joint arthrodesis. They reported a 100% bony fusion rate and a satisfactory result in 59 of 62 toes.

COMPLICATIONS

Hammer-toe correction with PIP joint resection arthroplasty or fusion is a generally successful and safe procedure with low rates of reported major complications in multiple series.[5–8] Reported complications include

- Pin tract infection
- Pin migration or breakage
- Malalignment
- Recurrent deformity
- Iatrogenic mallet toe deformity
- Instability
- Toe swelling
- Vascular insult causing toe necrosis

In Coughlin and colleagues' series, 10% of patients experienced a perioperative complication. Complications included superficial surgical site infections that were successfully treated with oral antibiotics (5% of patients), K-wire extrusions (1.5% of patients), and vascular insults that required early pin removal (3% of patients). Long-term complications included the recurrence of hammer toe (6% of toes), iatrogenic mallet toe (8% of toes), and postoperative numbness (6% of toes). One toe (1 of 118 toes, <1% of toes) went on the necessitate amputation. The reported malalignment rate was 15%, but most of these deformities were considered minor. Malalignment and postoperative numbness were the most-cited reasons for patient dissatisfaction.[5]

In 2015, Kramer and colleagues[8] reported complication rates in a very large series of hammer-toe corrections with K-wire fixation. This series included 2698 toes with an average follow-up of 20.8 months. K-wires were left in place for an average of 39.2 days. The reported complications included

- Pin migration (3.5%)
- Pin tract infection (0.3%)
- Pin breakage (0.1%)
- Recurrent deformities (5.6%)
- Revision surgery (3.5%)
- Malalignment (2.1%)
- Vascular compromise (0.6%)
- Amputation of toe (0.4%)

In Kramer and colleagues'[8] series, revision surgery was significantly more likely in patients who underwent concurrent MTP joint capsulotomy (relative risk [RR] = 3.2) indicating possibly more severe deformities than in those who had K-wire–associated complications (RR = 2.87). These more recent studies demonstrate relatively low K-wire–associated complication rates and somewhat contrast the classically cited series presented by Reece and associates.[9] In their retrospective study, an 18% infection rate was noted with percutaneous K-wire fixation when wires were left in place for 6 weeks.

Klammer and associates[7] conducted a randomized controlled trial comparing 3 weeks versus 6 weeks of K-wire fixation following PIP joint resection arthroplasty. They compared complication rates and alignment at a short-term follow-up of 3 months. They noted no statistical difference between the groups with regard to change in AOFAS score, infection rates, or pin-associated complications; however, they did note early postoperative malalignment in 47.8% versus 8.7% of toes pinned for 3 weeks versus 6 weeks, respectively.[7]

ALTERNATIVE FIXATION METHODS

Although K-wire fixation has historically been considered the standard for stabilization of the PIP joint in hammer-toe correction, many other forms of intramedullary fixation have been shown to be safe and effective while avoiding some of the potential complications associated with the presence of an exposed temporary implant.[10] Other forms of fixation include (**Fig. 5**)

- Cannulated screws
- Headless compression screws
- 1-piece intramedullary implants
- 2-piece intramedullary implants
- Nitinol shape memory intramedullary implants
- Absorbable intramedullary implants
- Allograft bone dowels

Caterini and associates[11] evaluated PIP joint fusion with intramedullary cannulated screws for hammer-toe correction. In their series of 51 toes in 24 patients, a 94% fusion rate was reported at the 1- to 4-year follow-up. Complete pain relief was reported in 79% of patients, and unqualified patient satisfaction was reported in 83% of cases. There was one broken screw and one surgical site infection that necessitated hardware removal. An additional 5 screws were removed secondary to persistent pain at the tip of the toe. Patients were allowed to begin normal shoe wear at 2 weeks postoperatively, which would not be possible with temporary K-wire fixation. The investigators note that no iatrogenic mallet toes developed, which is one potential benefit of an implant that crosses both the PIP and DIP joints.[11] This same consideration is often cited as a drawback of cannulated screw fixation because the DIP joint may not be involved in the hammer-toe deformity.

Coillard and colleagues[12] published a prospective multicenter study in 2014 evaluating a one-piece permanent intramedullary implant (Ipp-on, Integra Lifesciences Services, France) for the stabilization of the PIP joint in lesser-toe deformities. The study included 156 toes in 117 patients with 12 months of follow-up. Radiographic union was observed in 84% of toes. Complete resolution of pain was noted in 95% of patients at 1 year, and patient satisfaction was achieved in 98% of cases. The overall

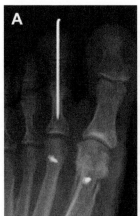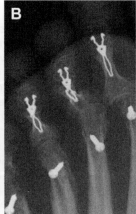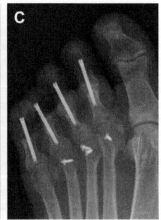

Fig. 5. Various types of fixation devices. (*A*) K-wire. (*B*) Nitinol permanent implant (Smart Toe, Stryker, Mahwah, NJ). (*C*) Cannulated screws.

complication rate was 4.5% and included 2 intraoperative fractures of the proximal phalanx, 3 instances of implant loosening, 1 broken implant, and only 1 reoperation within the 12-month follow-up period.[12]

Basile and associates[13] prospectively analyzed their results with another one-piece intramedullary device (PRO-TOE, Wright Medical Group, Memphis, TN) in the treatment of hammer-toe deformities. In this series of 60 rigid hammer toes with an 18-month follow-up, they observed a union rate of 85.0% with complete resolution of preoperative symptoms in 86.2% of patients. Their reported complication rate was low, with only 1 implant-related complication that required revision surgery. One hundred percent of patients stated that they would undergo the procedure again.[13]

Ellington and colleagues[14] reported their experience with a 2-piece intramedullary device (Stayfuse, Zimmer Inc, USA) in a retrospective series of 38 toes that included 26 revision hammer-toe procedures for recurrent deformity. They reported a union rate of 60.5% and an overall maintenance of coronal and sagittal alignment of 81.6% at an average of 31 months of follow-up. There were no reoperations in the primary repair group; however, the reoperation rate was 11.6% in the revision group.[14]

Jay and associates[15] conducted a randomized controlled clinical trial comparing outcomes and complication rates between a 2-piece intramedullary implant (Nextra, Nextremity Solutions, Inc, Warsaw, IN) and K-wire fixation for proximal interphalangeal joint fusion. At the 6-month follow-up, there was no difference in complication rates. The radiographic fusion rates were 16% and 84% for K-wire and intramedullary device fixation, respectively. Foot function index scores improved in both groups, but there was a trend toward greater improvement in outcome scores in the intramedullary device group.[15]

Nitinol memory-metal implants are uniquely designed to change shape in response to temperature changes. These types of implants are stored at cooler temperatures; once implanted, they expand in width and shorten in length to provide both improved fixation and compression at the anticipated fusion site.[16]

Catena and associates[16] prospectively evaluated hammer-toe deformities treated with PIP joint fusion using a nitinol memory-metal intramedullary implant (Smart Toe, Stryker, Mahwah, NJ) and a temporary K-wire. There were 43 toes (24 patients) with an average 12-month follow-up. They observed an 81% bony union rate and 100% patient satisfaction. Complication rates were low with 5% superficial infections, 5% skin edge necrosis, no cases of transverse plane malalignment, and no need for revision or secondary surgical procedures.[16]

Konkel and associates[17] reported on their series of 47 toes (29 patients) that underwent hammer-toe correction with poly-L-lactate absorbable pin fixation. At an average of 18 months of follow-up, they noted an 83.0% fusion rate; 96.5% of patients were satisfied with the procedure, and 93.0% of patients stated that they would undergo the procedure again. Only 1 infection was reported, and this was successfully treated with oral antibiotics. There were no cases of transverse plane malalignment.[17]

Although there is not an overwhelming body of evidence to support that permanent intramedullary fixation devices are superior to K-wire fixation in PIP joint fusion for hammer-toe deformity correction, multiple series demonstrate that these devices are often efficacious and safe with high rates of patient satisfaction. Further evaluation is needed to determine the cost-effectiveness of these devices in addition to outcomes when compared with K-wire fixation. The authors' preferred technique uses temporary K-wire fixation in the setting of primary hammer-toe correction, and a cannulated headless compression screw is preferred for the treatment of recurrent hammer-toe deformities.

SUMMARY

Hammer-toe deformities that fail nonoperative treatment can be successfully addressed with PIP joint resection arthroplasty or fusion. The goal of surgery is to rigidly fix the joint in a well-aligned position. This repair can be achieved by both bony fusion or fibrous union that leads to ankylosis of the joint.[5]

Hammer-toe correction procedures performed with temporary K-wire fixation for 3 to 6 weeks are highly successful. Complications seem to be exceedingly rare in most series, but there remains a concern regarding exposed temporary K-wire fixation. This concern has led to the development of multiple permanent internal fixation options. A review of the literature suggests that many of these permanent implants are both safe and effective. There may be some additional benefit to the utilization of permanent implants for revision hammer-toe surgery.

REFERENCES

1. Coughlin MJ, Saltzman CL, Anderson RB. Mann's surgery of the foot and ankle. 9th edition. Philadelphia: Elsevier Inc; 2014.
2. Taylor RG. The treatment of claw toes by multiple tendon transfers of flexor into extensor tendons. J Bone Joint Surg Br 1951;33:539–42.
3. Ellington JK. Hammertoes and claw toes: proximal interphalangeal joint correction. Foot Ankle Clin 2011;16:547–58.
4. Shirzad K, Kiesau C, DeOrio J, et al. Lesser toe deformities. J Am Acad Orthop Surg 2011;19(8):505–14.
5. Coughlin MJ, Dorris J, Polk E. Operative repair of the fixed hammertoe deformity. Foot Ankle Int 2000;21:94–104.
6. Ohm OW II, Mcdonell M, Vetter WA. Digital arthrodesis: an alternate method for correction of hammer toe deformity. J Foot Surg 1990;29:207–11.
7. Klammer G, Baumann G, Beat K. Early complications and recurrence rates after Kirschner wire transfixion in lesser toe surgery: a prospective randomized study. Foot Ankle Int 2012;33:105–12.
8. Kramer W, Parman M, Marks R. Hammertoe correction with k-wire fixation. Foot Ankle Int 2015;36(5):494–502.
9. Reece AT, Stone MH, Young AB. Toe fusion using Kirschner wire. A study of the postoperative infection rate and related problems. J R Coll Surg Edinb 1987; 32(3):158–9.
10. Guelfi M, Pantalone A, Daniel JC, et al. Arthrodesis of the proximal interphalangeal joint for hammertoe: intramedullary device options. J Orthop Traumatol 2015;16:269–73.
11. Caterini R, Farsetti P, Tarantino U, et al. Arthrodesis of the toe joints with an intramedullary cannulated screw for correction of hammertoe deformity. Foot Ankle Int 2004;25(4):256–61.
12. Coillard J, Petri GJ, Damme G, et al. Stabilization of proximal interphalangeal joint in lesser toe deformities with an angulated intramedullary implant. Foot Ankle Int 2014;35(4):401–7.
13. Basile A, Albo F, Via AG. Intramedullary fixation system for the treatment of hammertoe deformity. J Foot Ankle Surg 2015;54:910–6.
14. Ellington JK, Anderson R, Hodges D, et al. Radiographic analysis of proximal interphalangeal joint arthrodesis with an intramedullary fusion device for lesser toe deformities. Foot Ankle Int 2010;31(5):372–6.

15. Jay RM, Malay DS, Landsman A, et al. Dual-component intramedullary implant versus Kirschner wire for proximal interphalangeal joint fusion: a randomized controlled clinical trial. J Foot Ankle Surg 2016;55:697–708.
16. Catena F, Doty JF, Jastifer J, et al. Prospective study of hammertoe correction with an intramedullary implant. Foot Ankle Int 2014;35(4):319–25.
17. Konkel KF, Sover E, Menger A, et al. Hammer toe correction using an absorbable pin. Foot Ankle Int 2011;32(10):973–8.

Lesser Metatarsophalangeal Joint Instability: Treatment with Tendon Transfers

Caio Nery, MD[a],*, Daniel Baumfeld, MD[b]

KEYWORDS

- Tendon transfers • Forefoot deformities • Lesser toe instability
- Forefoot reconstruction • Plantar plate tear
- Metatarsophalangeal joints forefoot flexor tendon transfer

KEY POINTS

- Instability at the metatarsophalangeal joint of the lesser toes is challenging to treat, particularly when both transverse and sagittal plane deformity coexist.
- Indications for tendon transfer to treat lesser metatarsophalangeal joint instability are grade 4 plantar plate tears, in which the plantar plate and collateral ligaments cannot be restored.
- Tendon transfers for metatarsophalangeal joint deformities are just one surgical option for correction.
- Tendon transfers are usually not standalone procedures, and typically, a combination of procedures is needed for full correction.
- A tendon should be transferred under physiologic tension. If the tension is too tight, stiffness will result. If not enough tension is used, recurrence can result.

INTRODUCTION

Instability at the metatarsophalangeal (MTP) joint of the lesser toes is challenging to treat, particularly when both transverse and sagittal plane deformity coexist. In the last decade, there has been increasing interest in this pathology, particularly the involvement and importance of the plantar plate.[1–3] The plantar plate plays an important role in the stabilization of the lesser MTP joints, and some biomechanical studies demonstrated that the plantar plate is the main isolated stabilizer of the MTP joints in the dorsal–plantar direction.[4] Chalayon and colleagues[5] complemented the

Disclosure: Dr C. Nery is Speaker for Artrhex, Inc and Wright Med Tech, Inc, USA. Dr D. Baumfeld have no conflicts to disclose.
[a] UNIFESP - Federal University of São Paulo, R. Sena Madureira, 1500 - Vila Clementino, São Paulo - SP, 04021-001, Brazil; [b] UFMG - Federal University of Minas Gerais, Belo Horizonte, Av. Pres. Antônio Carlos, 6627 - Pampulha, Belo Horizonte - MG, 31270-901, Brazil
* Corresponding author.
E-mail address: caionerymd@gmail.com

biomechanical analysis of the lesser toes, evaluating stability of the MTP joint after sectioning the plantar plate in cadaveric specimens. Their results revealed significantly decreased stability in dorsiflexion, plantar flexion, and in dorsal translation. Barg and colleagues[6] described accessory collateral ligament tears leading to reductions of force to dorsally subluxate the lesser MTP joint.

Grading schemes describing MTP joint instability have been proposed. The main purposes of these grading systems are to address the pathophysiology of the lesions and to stratify different stages of soft tissue involvement, to create a treatment algorithm with alternatives for each different stage of MTP plantar plate lesion.[7–9]

Many studies addressed the treatment of advanced lesser toe deformities. However, most of them do not relate the deformities to plantar plate tears, and, if so, they do not differentiate and classify the many different patterns of the pathology.[10]

The rationale for using a tendon transfer to treat lesser MTP join instability is based on the premise that, when transferred, the tendon can substitute for the loss of intrinsic musculature function, restore stability, and improve the function of the lesser toes.[11] In our opinion, tendon transfers are reliable options to approach the lesser MTP joint instability only when the main stabilizers of the joint cannot be repaired.

PATIENT ASSESSMENT

As with any encounter with a patient, a thorough history and physical examination is essential. It is important to take note of a history of previous trauma or surgery, because this finding may change the morphology of the foot. The examination begins with observation of gait and any obvious deformities. The patient is examined in the seated and standing positions. Assessment of foot shape and associated deformities (hallux valgus or rigidus) is documented. One should also evaluate toes misalignments in different planes: axial (varus/valgus), frontal (supination/pronation), and sagittal (dorsal/plantar), the ability of the toe to touch the ground, the strength of the toe purchase and joint instability (**Fig. 1**).

Clinical observation and physical examinations should be performed carefully and graded using the clinical staging system, which has good correlation with intraoperative findings.[12] A lesser MTP drawer test is one of the most important tests that helps to grade the amount of instability.[13,14] Digital toe purchase is used to analyze the balance and function of the muscles across the lesser MTP joint.

It is often helpful to have the patient point to the area of maximal tenderness. Calluses or keratosis may be localized under a particular metatarsal or may be more diffuse in nature. In addition to visual inspection, a neurovascular examination is performed.

Assessment of the gastroc soleus tightness is paramount and is done by performing the Silfverskiold test.[15]

Palpation of the web space between the metatarsal heads as well as the Mulder's test is strongly recommended. Pain elicited with these maneuver suggests interdigital neuritis or Morton's neuroma (**Fig. 2**).

Anteroposterior, lateral, and oblique weight bearing comparative plain radiographs are necessary to evaluate the MTP joint and exclude osseous pathology. The anteroposterior weight bearing views can demonstrate second metatarsal pathologic excessive length (MT head protrusion), altered metatarsal parabola, splaying of the affected and adjacent toe or a subluxated toe with overlapping between the phalanx and the metatarsal.

Lateral weight bearing radiographs can demonstrate a toe elevation with the proximal phalanx lying dorsally at the metatarsal head[12] (**Fig. 3**).

MRI can be used to help in decision making between plantar plate reconstruction or tendon transfer.[16] This study can show an eccentric pericapsular soft tissue

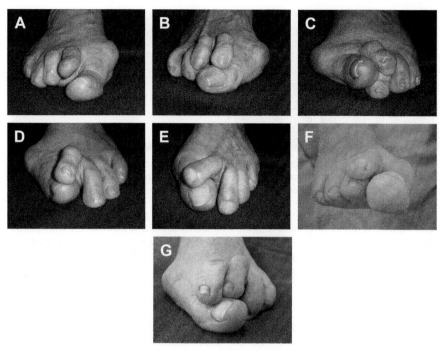

Fig. 1. Lesser toe deformities. (*A*) Second toe elevated and mildly supinated and superimposed to the great toe. (*B*) Claw toes with second and third crossing over the great toe. (*C*) Second hammertoe with valgus and pronation superimposed to the third claw toe. (*D*) Classic crossover second toe with varus and supination deformity combined with dorsal proximal interphalangeal hyperkeratosis. (*E*) Crossover of the second toe with varus and gross supination. (*F*) Second pronated toe crossing over the third toe. (*G*) Crossing over of the second and third toes with no rotational deformities.

thickening, increase of lesser metatarsal supination, and rupture of the plantar plate in sagittal and coronal images. There are reproducible differences in the measurement of metatarsal axis rotation and second metatarsal protrusion and their relation with plantar plate tears. Lesser metatarsal supination of greater than 36° or second

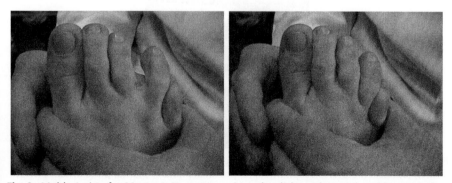

Fig. 2. Mulder's sign for Morton's Neuroma: pain and a click can be produced by squeezing the forefoot with 1 hand while some pressure is applied in the sole of the foot (at the level of the intermetatarsal space to be examined) with the thumb of the other hand.

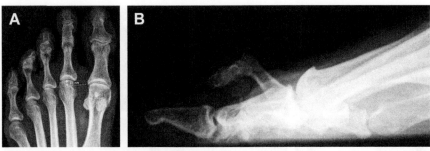

Fig. 3. (A) Protrusion of the second metatarsal head (anteroposterior weight bearing view). (B) Intense elevation of the second toe (lateral weight bearing view) with dorsal dislocation of the metatarsophalangeal joint.

metatarsal protrusion of greater than 4 mm trend toward a correlation with plantar plate tear. Lesser metatarsal supination of less than 24° is a strong negative predictor, and second metatarsal protrusion of greater than 4.5 mm is a strong positive predictor of plantar plate tear[17] (**Fig. 4**).

CLASSIFICATION

Although several grading schemes for describing second MTP joint instability have been described,[7,18–20] we now use a comprehensive clinical staging system

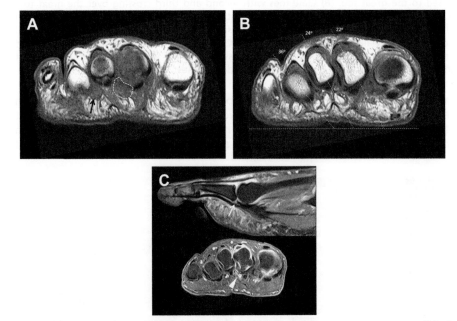

Fig. 4. (A) Pericapsular soft tissue thickening (*dotted shape*). Morton's neuroma (*black arrow*), (B) lesser metatarsals supination, (C) proximal phalanx–plantar plate distance (*white arrow*) and longitudinal plantar plate tears are important MRI signals correlated with metatarsophalangeal plantar plate tears. At the coronal plane, longitudinal tears can be detected (*white arrowhead*).

(Appendix 1) based on the physical examination findings that incorporates many of the principles of previous rating systems.[9] An anatomic grading system to accompany the staging system has been developed from the findings from the dissection of cadaveric specimens with plantar plate pathologic features. These systems address plantar plate dysfunction and are helpful in quantifying the magnitude of the deformity and guide preoperative planning for surgical repair. Nery and colleagues[12] reported on a series of 55 plantar plate tears evaluated arthroscopically before open repair and found that a grade 3 tear was most common and accounted for almost one-half of all the tears. This same author has reported that the previous knowledge of the anatomic grading system helps the radiologist find and describe the plantar plate tear and the degrees of lesser MTP joint instability.

DECISION MAKING

Tendon transfers are just 1 option that can be added to the procedure selection for digital and MTP joint deformities, and they are not typically performed as standalone procedures.[21] Usually, a combination of osseous and soft tissue procedures is necessary to gain adequate correction of the deformity. A stepwise approach should be used to thoroughly evaluate the deformity, address all deforming forces, and devise an appropriate treatment regimen. Experience demonstrates that these deformities are not the same and cannot be treated as such. What may work on 1 deformity may not work on another.

Because there is no gold standard for all digital deformities, it may be difficult to clearly define the absolute indication for the tendon transfer. It may be used for a variety of situations and in combination with additional procedures. It is best considered as a useful adjunct if the main stabilizer of the joint cannot be repaired.

Using the anatomic classification,[22] indications for tendon transfer to treat lesser MTP joint instability include grade 4 plantar plate tears. In this situation, plantar plate and collateral ligaments cannot be restored.

SURGICAL TREATMENT
Preoperative Discussion

This type of treatment involves a meticulous forefoot reconstruction and the patient must understand that the main objective is pain relief and improve shoe wear. Sometimes, a perfect toe alignment and full range of motion is not possible to achieve. The possibility of wound breakdown, deep surgical site infection, and painful scarring of the dorsum of the foot should be discussed as well. Reconstruction results are reasonable, but by no means perfect.[11,23] The vascular status of the foot must be excellent, and the patient should stop smoking at least for 14 days before the surgery.

PATIENT POSITION AND INCISIONS

The patient is positioned supine with the feet at the distal border of the operative table. The surgical bed can be elevated in a Trendelenburg position if the surgeon needs access to the plantar aspect of the foot. To avoid external rotation of the foot one can use a small pad under the back of the patient. Anesthesia is usually intravenous sedation with local infiltrative or spinal blocks. An Esmarch elastic wrap or ankle tourniquet can be used to control surgical bleeding and increase visualization.

The surgeon starts the procedure facing the dorsal aspect of the forefoot while the first assistant faces the sole of the foot. In some steps of the procedure, they will change their positions to make the surgical maneuvers feasible. The MTP joint is approached through a standard dorsal longitudinal incision 3 to 4 cm over the dorsum of the joint.[24] If more than 1 MTP joint will be accessed, the incision can be placed between the metatarsal heads or an "S"-shaped incision can be used[25] (**Fig. 5**).

The incision is deepened in the space between the extensor digitorum longus (EDL) and brevis (EDB), protecting the vascular supply structures. A dorsal longitudinal MTP capsulotomy is performed followed by a partial collateral ligament release (medially and/or laterally, depending on the grade and orientation of the deformity) of the proximal phalanx. Plantar-flexing the toe at the MTP joint helps to complete the soft tissue release. In the case of persistent deformity, a McGlamry elevator can help to expose the plantar plate and release all inflammatory adhesions without compromising the local vascular supply.

METATARSAL OSTEOTOMY

The most common initial operative approach for second MPJ instability involves soft tissue rebalancing with various capsulotomies and metatarsal osteotomies. Bone procedures have the objective of realigning the metatarsal parabola, decompressing the MTP joint, and allowing the reduction of the subluxated joint. As described by Maestro and colleagues,[26] the need for some degree of metatarsal shortening may be judged based on the harmonious forefoot morphotype.

The Weil procedure has been popularized to treat this pathology because of its simplicity, ease of fixation, and relative stability, but this procedure can potentially lead to a postoperative floating toe deformity.[10,27] A floating toe deformity can be defined as a lack of digital purchase during the stance phase of gait.[10] Multiple theories have been suggested in the literature as to the possible causes of the

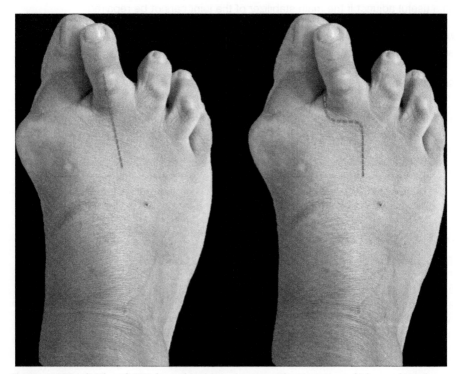

Fig. 5. Longitudinal and "S"-shaped incisions to access the metatarsophalangeal joint.

postoperative floating toe. The most accepted are the absence of reconstruction of the primary stabilizer of the joint (plantar plate and collateral ligaments) and the changes in the center of rotation of the MTP joint axis after the osteotomy. For this reason, these authors do not recommend the use of this osteotomy alone; it must be a part of a complete joint reconstruction.

Technique

A Weil distal metatarsal osteotomy is performed using a sagittal saw (**Fig. 6**). The saw cut is made parallel to the plantar aspect of the foot, starting at a point 2 to 3 mm below the top of the metatarsal articular surface. Keeping the osteotomy as parallel as possible with the sole is paramount owing to the plantar declination of the metatarsal and to avoid the plantar aspect of the metatarsal head articular surface. In the presence of a plantar keratosis beneath the metatarsal head, a small slice of bone can be removed to achieve a subtle elevation of the metatarsal head. Pay attention not to shorten the metatarsal that is greater than 3 mm (see **Fig. 6**).

TENDON TRANSFER

Tendon transfers are important tools for a variety of purposes in forefoot deformity. They allow for the correction of deformity, establishment or augmentation of motor function, or the generation of a tenodesis effect.

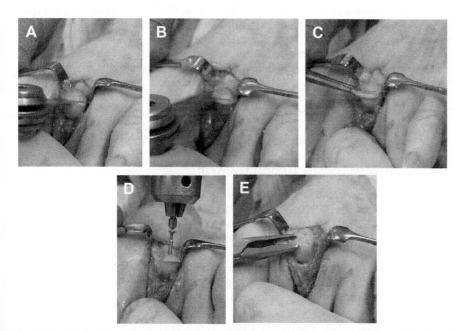

Fig. 6. The Weil osteotomy. (*A*) The entry point of the saw is 2 to 3 mm distal to the dorsal border of the metatarsal head articular surface. The orientation of the cut must be as parallel as possible with the ground plane. (*B*) In the presence of metatarsalgia, in which some elevation of the metatarsal head is necessary, a second cut can be done, parallel to the first cut, to remove a 1-mm slice of bone of the metatarsal head–neck region. (*C*) The bone slice is removed. (*D*) Keeping the metatarsal head in the desired position, a snap-off screw is used to fix the osteotomy. (*E*) The overhanging portion of the dorsal metatarsal metaphysis is removed to recreate a round metatarsal head.

Some prerequisites are needed for successful tendon transfer[21]:

- Analysis of the patient's needs and goals.
- Knowledge of the patient's appreciation of surgical expectations and limitations.
- Adequate soft tissue bed for coverage.
- Mobile intercalary joints.
- Donor motor unit that has adequate strength, sufficient excursion, and expendability.

Once these prerequisites have been met, there are basic principles that the surgeon should use to decide on the best motor unit to transfer for balance between the transferred tendon and its opposing muscles.[21,28]

Basic Principles of Successful Tendon Transfer

- Appropriate strength.
- Appropriate amplitude.
- Direction and attachment.
- Synergy and phase of muscle transfer.
- Integrity.
- Tensioning.
- Formation of a stable bone–tendon interface.

The key factor of tendon transfer for subluxated MTP joint is the attenuation and rupture of the plantar plate and collateral ligaments. Without the possibility of repair of the main stabilizer of the joint, tendon transfer is a viable option in conjunction with metatarsal osteotomy.[29]

Tendon transfer techniques attempt to supplement for the deficient plantar plate while counterbalancing the tendon deformation. Transferring tendon has the objective to replace the loss of intrinsic muscular function and help to rebalance the deformity, especially deviations in the coronal plane.

There are 2 groups of tendons that can be transferred at the MTP joint, the flexor tendons and the extensor tendons.[30] Recently, the use of synthetic material for free grafts has been described in the literature as alternative option.[31]

FLEXOR DIGITORUM LONGUS TENDON TRANSFER

The rationale for use of a flexor-to-extensor transfer is based on the premise that the flexor digitorum longus (FDL) tendon, when transferred to the dorsum of the proximal phalanx, can substitute for lost intrinsic function (flexion at the MTP joint and resistance to extension at the interphalangeal joints), and toe mechanics are, therefore, restored. The deforming force of the FDL tendon and the release of the extensor tendon also play important roles in correcting the deformity.[11,32]

There are multiple approaches for this specific tendon transfer, depending on other procedures being concomitantly performed, the severity and complexity of the deformity, and surgeon preference.

Because of unfavorable results, it is not common to perform the FDL tendon transfer as a standalone procedure.[33] Typically, this procedure is done in conjunction with metatarsal osteotomy and, in some cases, with a proximal interphalangeal joint arthrodesis and with flexor tendon lengthening. We believe that this procedure is appropriate for both flexible and rigid lesser toe deformity. For a lasting correction to be achieved, it must not only correct the existing anatomic deficiency, but also in some fashion alter the biomechanical tendency that caused the plantar plate to rupture in the first place.[11]

Technique

This procedure can be performed with a 1-, 2-, or 3-incision technique.[23,32] The 3-incision technique is the most common used and describe as follows (**Fig. 7**).

- Transverse incision on the plantar aspect of the toe, at the level of the distal interphalangeal joint. The flexor tendon is released from its insertion at the inferior border of the distal phalanx.
- Another transverse incision at the level of the proximal digital plantar crease is used to dissect and isolate the FDL tendon at the flexor's tunnel.
- The tendon is isolated from the split flexor digitorum brevis tendon using a hemostat.
- The tendon is pulled proximal and transected. The tendon is split into equal halves. Each half is clamped with a hemostat.
- Through a dorsal incision centered over the proximal phalanx, the tails of the FDL are passed at the medial and lateral aspect of the extensor hood in the midportion of the proximal phalanx. The subcutaneous tissues are divided in line with the skin incision, with care taken to limit dissection laterally to avoid neurovascular injury.
- With the toe placed in 20° of plantar flexion of the MTP joint, the flexor tendons were sutured to the extensor hood under a slight degree of tension.
- The tendon complex is then sutured into the EDL.
- After, routine wound closure.

Two-Incision Technique

The 2-incision approach follows the same sequence described for the 3-incision technique; the main difference is a longitudinal plantar incision over the affected digit instead of 2 transversal plantar incisions (**Fig. 8**).[23]

Another possibility is to place the incision lateral and medial in the toe:

- One incision is made on the side of the toe, typically medially on the second toe and lateral on the third, fourth, and fifth toes, to provide the greatest exposure.
- Sharp dissection is performed to open the retinacula binding the flexor tendons to the underside of the phalanges. The FDL tendon is severed distally near its attachment at the base of the distal phalanx.
- The longus tendon is then split longitudinally to the base of the proximal phalanx. A second incision is made dorsally and opposite the side of the initial incision on the proximal phalanx.
- A channel is created medially and laterally around the bone with a periosteal elevator, and then the tendon slips are drawn dorsally around the proximal phalanx and sutured upon themselves with nonabsorbable suture.

One-Incision Technique

When performing a concomitant rigid hammertoe repair with the flexor tendon transfer, the FDL tendon can be identified easily through the dorsal incision of the toe at the level of the proximal interphalangeal joint. With this approach, the technique can be performed through the dorsal incision only.[23,34,35]

- A central dorsolinear incision is made from middle phalanx extending proximally to the MTP joint.
- The incision can be curved over the MTP joint.
- The subcutaneous tissues are reflected, avoiding the neurovascular bundles medially and laterally.

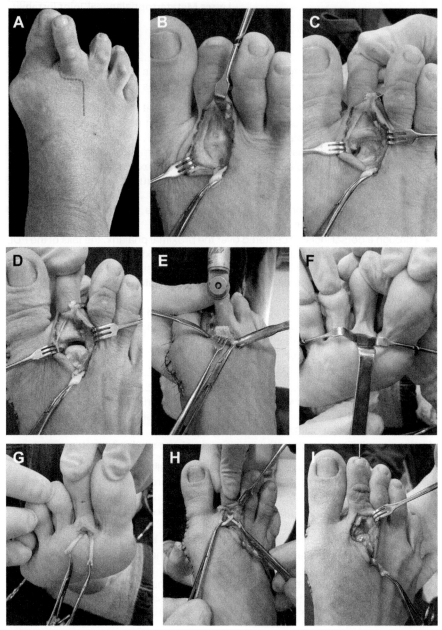

Fig. 7. Flexor digitorum longus (FDL) tendon transfer technique (3-incision approach). (*A*) A long dorsal "S"-shaped incision is advisable in the presence of a crossover toe deformity with subluxation or dislocation of the metatarsophalangeal (MTP) joint. (*B*) The extensor tendons are lengthened when necessary and the dorsal MTP joint capsule is exposed. (*C*, *D*) Proper and accessory collateral ligaments are sectioned to achieve alignment of the articular surfaces. (*E*) A Weil osteotomy is often required to correct the metatarsal parabola and to reduce the plantar overloading of the metatarsal head. (*F*) Through a transverse small incision at the base of the toe, the flexor tendon's tunnel is dissected. The central 2 bands of tendon found there corresponds with the FDL tendon and they are isolated with a hemostat. (*G*) A second plantar transverse incision at the level of the distal interphalangeal joint is made to release the FDL insertion at the base of the distal phalanx. Both halves are exteriorized through the proximal incision. (*H*) The 2 bands of the FDL are passed, medially and

A   **B**

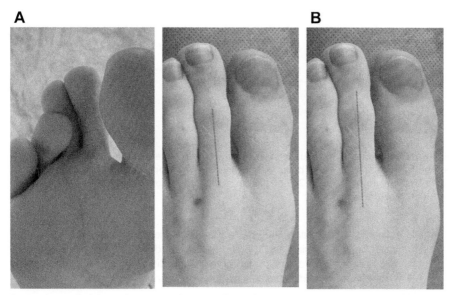

Fig. 8. Flexor digitorum longus tendon transfer technique. (*A*) A 2-incision approach. (*B*) A 1-incision approach.

- The extensor expansion is incised medially and laterally, and either a transverse tenotomy or lengthening of the extensor tendon is performed.
- Attention is then directed back to the proximal interphalangeal joint, where the medial and lateral collateral ligaments are incised to expose the joint. If a proximal interphalangeal joint arthrodesis or arthroplasty is performed, the joint is prepared as per surgeon preference.
- The plantar tissue of the proximal interphalangeal joint is incised at the base of the middle phalanx. At this level, the FDL tendon will be located centrally between the tendon slips of the flexor digitorum brevis.
- The FDL tendon is then isolated and transected within the proximal interphalangeal joint.
- Each of the tendon halves is then transferred proximally and dorsally around the proximal phalanx.
- The proximal interphalangeal joint is fixated, using the surgeons' preferred method.
- The FDL tendon halves are then brought dorsally over the proximal phalanx and sutured together, typically with 3-0 nonabsorbable sutures, under appropriate tension.

Alternative Transfer Method and Tendon Fixation

Instead of splitting the FDL tendon and passing the 2 sleeves medial and lateral around the proximal phalanx, one can use a bone tunnel to move the tendon from plantar to dorsal[36,37] (**Fig. 9**).

laterally, from plantar to dorsal and are sutured at the extensor hood while the toe is kept in 20° of flexion. (*I*) As a complementary procedure, resection arthroplasty of the proximal interphalangeal joint (DuVries) have to be considered to achieve a good correction. K-wire fixation is advisable, especially in younger patients; the extensor tendons are sutured at the appropriate length and a careful hemostasis is done before skin closure.

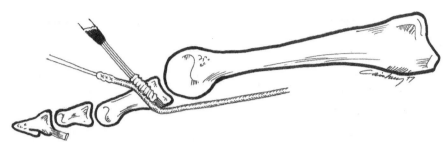

Fig. 9. Flexor digitorum longus tendon transfer: alternative technique using a bone hole at the base of the proximal phalanx and a small biotenodesis screw to fix the tendon. Note that the toe is kept in 20° of flexion during this procedure to achieve the correct tensioning of the tendon.

- When using this approach, the FDL tendon is transected at the level of the proximal interphalangeal joint, and a drill hole is placed in the base of the proximal phalanx directed from dorsal proximal to plantar distal.
- A wire loop can be used to pull the tendon from plantar to dorsal through the drill hole.
- Bone anchors or a small biotenodesis screw can be used to secure the tendon in the dorsal phalanx.

EXTENSOR DIGITORUM TENDONS TRANSFER

Extensor tendons transfer has been described as alternatives to flexor-to-extensor transfer in the treatment of lesser MTP joint instability in an effort to avoid postoperative complications and patient dissatisfaction related to those procedures.[38] This procedure can be performed with the EDL or the EDB, both located dorsally of the MTP joint and easily accessed during the exposure of this joint.

EXTENSOR DIGITORUM LONGUS TENDON TRANSFER

In 2004, Barca and Acciaro[39] described a new technique for transfer of the EDL tendon to treat the crossover toe deformity. After releasing all soft tissue contractures around the affected MTP joint, the EDL is sectioned at the level of the proximal interphalangeal joint, leaving the EDB intact. The proximal portion of the tendon is then passed under the deep intermetatarsal ligament lateral to the toe and driven from plantar lateral to medial dorsal into a bone tunnel made at the base of the proximal phalanx. The transferred tendon is kept in place with the help of a pull-out suture (button technique). Originally, the authors stabilized the MTP joint with a K-wire for 4 weeks (**Fig. 10**). They performed this technique on 30 toes and reported that 83% of the patients had excellent or good results (excellent in 10 toes and good in 15 toes).

Lui and Chan[40] have described a modification of the EDL tendon transfer technique. In this alternative technique, the extra length of the tendon is required to achieve a side-to-side anastomosis and create a better route for the transfer by passing the tendon through a drill hole in the base of the proximal phalanx.

Technique

- The surgical approach is similar with the dorsal incision previously described. The authors suggest extending the incision 5 cm proximal to the MP joint.

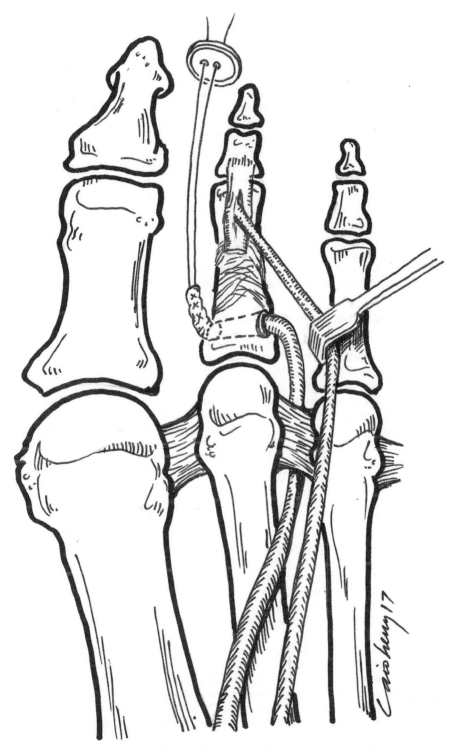

Fig. 10. Barca and Acciaro's technique for the transfer of the extensor digitorum longus tendon. See the text for details.

- The EDL tendon is lengthened in a standard Z-lengthening technique, the lengthening is done through very long limbs.
- The EDB tendon is sectioned as proximal to the metatarsal neck level as possible, creating a long distal cable to be sutured to the EDL proximal cable.
- The MP joint is addressed as necessary to address all soft tissue contractures.
- A transverse bone tunnel is made through the base of the proximal phalanx, just inferior to the midline of the phalanx. This tunnel should not be placed completely plantar, because that placement results in a hyperextension deformity of the MTP joint. As may be intuitive, if the tunnel is placed dorsal to the midline, a supination deformity will result. The ideal diameter of the tunnel is around 2.5 mm.
- The long distal limb of the EDL tendon is then passed, from medial to lateral, through the phalangeal bone tunnel. A tendon passer may be used, facilitated by a Krakow suture placed through the free end of the tendon.
- The same long distal limb of the EDL tendon is then passed from distal to proximal deep to the transverse metatarsal ligament and is sutured to the proximal stump of the EDB tendon.
- The EDL proximal limb is then sutured to the distal EDB limb.
- The authors suggest a K-wire fixation thought the MTP joint for 4 weeks (**Fig. 11**)

EXTENSOR DIGITORUM BREVIS TENDON TRANSFER

An EDB tendon transfer can also be performed for digital and MTP joint deformities. Haddad and colleagues[33] performed this procedure on 19 patients with a crossover second toe deformity. This analysis compared 16 patients with flexor-to-extensor tendon transfers and 19 patients with EDB tendon transfers and found that both treatment groups had similar results. Overall, 24 patients were completely satisfied; 6 patients had some minor reservations, and 1 patient was dissatisfied. The investigators did state, however, that, although most patients were free of pain at follow-up, those treated with the FDL tendon transfer tended to have more pain, and those with more pain had residual lack of motion at the MTP joint.

Technique

- A dorsal incision is made over the proximal phalanx and distal metatarsal of the affected digit.
- The EDB tendon and the EDL tendon are identified and followed proximally.
- Typically, a "Z"-lengthening of the EDL tendon is made, and the EDB is secured.
- Once the EDB is identified, a tenotomy is performed as proximal as possible, ideally just distal to the musculotendinous junction.
- It is important that the EDB is left intact at its distal attachment into the dorsal aspect of the proximal phalanx.
- Once the EDB is isolated and released proximally, sutures are applied to the tendon.
- At this point, a second MTP joint capsulotomy is performed and, depending on the nature of the deformity, collateral ligament, and/or plantar plate release and metatarsal osteotomy is performed as previously described.
- The transverse metatarsal ligament between the second and third metatarsal heads is defined. The distal EDB tendon is then passed from distal to proximal under the transverse intermetatarsal ligament on the convex side of the MTP coronal deformity.
- The EDB is then appropriately tensioned and secured to its proximal stump, with the coronal MTP deformity congruently corrected.

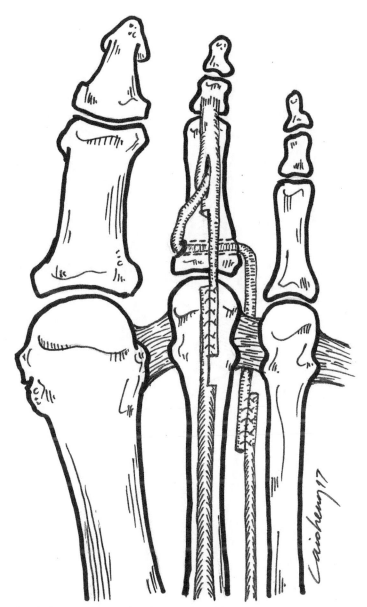

Fig. 11. Lui and Chan's technique for the transfer of the extensor digitorum longus tendon. See the text for details.

- These authors recommended the toe to be pinned across the MTP joint to secure the appropriated tension applied over the reconstruction.
- The K-wire is pulled out at 6 weeks (**Fig. 12**).

Alternative Extensor Digitorum Brevis Tendon Transfer

Commonly, the EDB transfer is performed as described, passing the tendon under the intermetatarsal ligament. Alternatively, bone tunnels can be created to guide the

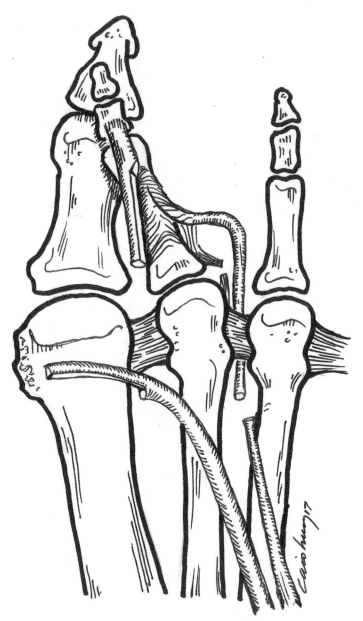

Fig. 12. Haddad and Myerson's technique for the transfer of extensor digitorum brevis tendon. See the text for details.

transferred tendon to correct the malalignment. Tunnels must be oriented according the deformities to be corrected. In the case of varus malalignment, the EDB is transferred to reconstruct the lateral collateral ligament. With a valgus deformity, the EDB is routed to mimic the medial collateral ligament. In the absence of a sagittal deformity, drill holes can be oriented transversely in the proximal phalanx and metatarsal head, parallel to the weight bearing surface. Drilling is performed medial to lateral in the proximal phalanx and lateral to medial in the metatarsal. If there is concomitant sagittal deformity, drill holes are oriented along an oblique dorsomedial to plantar–lateral axis.[41]

- The initial sequence is as described.
- After the EDB individualization, guidewire is placed in the proximal phalanx directed from dorsomedial to plantar–lateral.
- A second guidewire is placed in the metatarsal head, extending from the plantar–lateral corner of the articular surface to the dorsomedial metatarsal neck.
- Guidewire orientation is reversed in the event of a dorsiflexion/valgus deformity.
- The tendon diameter is measured; it is usually 2 or 3 mm.
- The tendon is then transferred through the bone tunnel with the use of tendon passer or wire loop. First, the tendon is passed through the base of the phalanx.
- The tendon exits the phalanx plantarly and then is routed from plantar to dorsal through the metatarsal bone tunnel.
- The fixation can be achieve with 3.0-mm biotenodesis screw or bone anchors.
- Digital alignment is then confirmed by intraoperative fluoroscopy.

OTHERS TYPES OF TENDON TRANSFERS
Synthetic Implants as Substitutes to Tendon Transfers for Metatarsophalangeal Joint Instability

Sung[31] in 2015 describe the use of a resistant synthetic tape along with 2 interference screws to address lesser MTP joint instability with grossly unstable or attenuated periarticular ligaments, especially when the plantar plate has been completely torn or is absent. The author advocate the use of this technique as an alternative to flexor tendon transfer in the presence of gross lesser MTP joint ligament instability, pain, and deformity owing to the absence of the plantar plate.[31]

Technique

- The dissection is initiated with an incision over the lesser MTP joint, and sharp dissection is carried subcutaneously to expose the target metatarsal head.
- A linear incision is then made to split the interval between the EDL and EDB tendons.
- A small McGlamry elevator is used to free the soft tissue attachments between the second metatarsal head and plantar plate.
- A 3.5-mm SwiveLock Suture Anchor (Arthrex Inc, Naples, FL) is seated in the metatarsal head. It is important to ensure that the eyelet in the anchor has been removed, making the 3.5-mm diameter anchor 8 mm in length.
- After, a 2-mm-wide, 7-inch-long FiberTape (Arthrex Inc) is passed through the channel in the metatarsal head using a suture passer and prepared for transfer through the MTP joint en route to the proximal phalangeal base.
- The proximal end of the tape is then secured using a 3.5-mm SwiveLock interference screw.
- The phalanx guidewire is then directed centrally from dorsally and distally to plantarly and proximally through the proximal phalangeal base, beginning at least 5 mm distal to the proximal margin of the base and exiting the plantar aspect just distal to the joint line.
- Thereafter, the tape is passed from plantarly and proximally to dorsally and distally through the phalanx and the tension is assessed by pressing a flat plate against the foot to visualize the toe and joint alignment.

- The tape should be tensioned to allow 10° to 15° of dorsiflexion in the sagittal plane or until toe purchase has been achieved.
- After satisfactory tension has been achieved, the eyelet is removed and the second 3.5-mm interference screw is positioned in the proximal phalanx.
- This procedure can be combined with metatarsal osteotomy, interphalangeal arthrodesis, or arthroplasty, as needed.
- If desired, a K-wire can be used to temporarily transfixate the MTP joint.
- After completion, the wound is closed in anatomic layers using sutures of the surgeon's choice (**Fig. 13**).

POSTOPERATIVE CARE

After surgery of the lesser toes, patients are allowed to ambulate in postoperative shoes for 4 to 6 weeks with no weight bearing on the forefoot with the toe taped in neutral or held in plantar flexion (**Fig. 14**). Dressings were discontinued and comfortable shoes were permitted after 4 to 6 weeks after surgery. An exercise program is then initiated to condition the extrinsic flexors of the lesser toes. If a K-wire was used to hold the toe in the desire position, it should be removed after 4 to 6 weeks.

COMPLICATIONS

The most common complications regarding the FDL tendon transfer are stiffness and residual and persistent swelling of the toe. Some stiffness, however, is believed to help reduce the risk of recurrence of deformity. In the same way, stiffness, swelling, residual pain, and recurrent deformity may complicate the postoperative course of patients who undergo EDB or EDL transfer.[23,42,43] Avoiding tendon transfer in patients with rigid deformities, evidence of interdigital neuroma, or both may minimize the chances of unsatisfactory outcomes.

Angular deformities, floating toe, lack of toe purchase, prolonged edema, scarring, numbness, and vascular insult can also occur after tendon transfers. Other complications include loss of active flexion, fracture of the proximal phalanx and metatarsal when using bone tunnels, screws, or anchors, and vascular impairments. The most serious complication of this kind of surgery occurs when the medial and lateral vascular bundles are damaged causing distal ischemia and necrosis that could end in partial or total amputation of the toe (**Fig. 15**).

It should be noted that the correction of very severe deformities, even in patients with normal peripheral circulation, can produce ischemia of the toes by stretching of the vessels. It is advisable to follow closely the vascularization of the digital pulp and the nail bed of these patients, especially when using K-wires in fixing the surgically obtained corrections. Sometimes, it is necessary to remove the K-wire immediately to avoid further soft tissue damage.

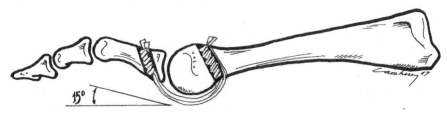

Fig. 13. Sung's technique. See the text for details.

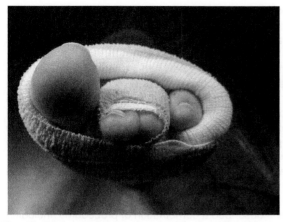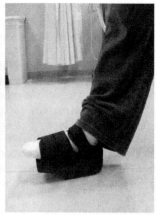

Fig. 14. Postoperative bandages with the affected toes kept in plantar 20° of plantar flexion and the Barouk's sandal used to protect the forefoot from weight bearing for 6 weeks.

CLINICAL RESULTS IN THE LITERATURE

Multiple methods for correction of gross MTP joint instability have been described. The Weil osteotomy technique and the flexor-to-extensor tendon transfer are the most common.[44] Few of these reports use some type of classification to stratify the grade of MTP instability. The literature is controversial regarding the FDL tendon transfer. Some surgeons avoid the procedure, stating that the toe becomes too stiff after the surgery; others, however, state that part of the success in the procedure is the stiffness it produces, because there is less chance of recurrence.[33,45,46]

The Weil osteotomy technique, on its own, has been one of the mainstays of surgical treatment for lesser MTP instability. In a prospective study with 7 years of follow-up, Hofstaetter and colleagues[10] found an 88% patient satisfaction rate. However, these

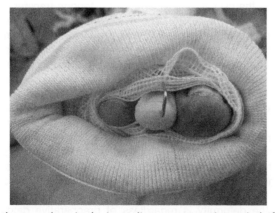

Fig. 15. Pallor of the second toe in the immediate postoperative period. If normalization of the peripheral circulation does not occur up to 20 minutes after releasing the pneumatic cuff, withdrawal of the K-wire and gradual return of the toe to the position of initial deformity is indicated.

authors demonstrated a 12% redislocation rate and a 68% incidence of floating toe. In a recent literature review, Highlander and colleagues[47] indicated that the floating toe was the most common complication of the Weil procedure, with a reported incidence average of 36%.

The other current option in the literature is the flexor-to-extensor transfer. Mendicino and colleagues[48] performed a retrospective analysis on 8 patients who underwent a flexor tendon transfer and had excellent results in 6 patients. Residual stiffness was the primary complaint of 2 patients after the procedure. Myerson and Jung[42] treated 64 feet with a split FDL tendon transfer and performed a retrospective analysis. Results included 26 patients who were satisfied, 15 patients who were satisfied with minor reservations, 6 patients who were satisfied with major reservations, and 12 patients who were not satisfied. Gazdag and Cracchiolo[19] reported 35% fair results in a series of 20 feet that were submitted to a flexor-to-extensor transfer.

In 2005, Shurnas and Sanders[36] described a combination of procedures, including oblique osteotomy of metatarsal, extensor lengthening with hammertoe repair, as well as flexor tendon transfer to the dorsal aspect of proximal phalanx fixated with a biotenodesis screw. They found excellent outcomes and minimal stiffness associated with this combination of procedures. This study did not use any anatomic or clinical classification to distinguish the degrees of deformities and its respective types of treatment.

The authors have an unpublished series of patients, all with grade 4 instability, who were treated with metatarsal osteotomy and flexor to extensor tendon transfer. This case series is different than the others in the literature because the degree of joint instability were the same in all patients. After a mean follow-up of 2 years, our results are promising. There were 88.2% congruent joints on postoperative radiographs, 47.1% of the joints with no elevation, and 100% of joints with improved stability and no major complications.

Iglesias and colleagues[46] performed a metaanalysis of the flexor tendon transfer with the aim of the study to evaluate the clinical benefit of the procedure. There were 203 articles retrieved; 17 publications met the inclusion criteria and were entered into the analysis. Overall patient satisfaction with the procedure was 86.7%. When adjusting for higher quality prospective studies, overall patient satisfaction was increased to 91.8%. These investigators concluded that there was supportive evidence of the clinical benefit of the FDL tendon transfer. They also found that there was no significant difference of success of the procedure regarding the age and sex of the patient. They further found that the most common reason for an unsatisfied patient was stiffness, and better satisfaction rates were found in toes that also had a proximal interphalangeal joint arthrodesis performed in addition to the tendon transfer.

The flexor digitorum brevis tendon has also been described to aid in stabilizing the MTP joint. Haddad and colleagues[33] reported their results with EDB tendon transfer. They noted a greater risk of recurrence with higher grade deformity. No relationship between the severity of the preoperative deformity and postoperative American Orthopedic Foot and Ankle Society score was observed. Marked improvement was seen in passive alignment and patient function. The EDB transfer represents an advance in the surgical treatment of lesser toe deformity. The reconstruction provides markedly improved control in the transverse plane and therefore has a role in the treatment of deformity where the deformity is regardless of preoperative deformity severity.[38] Furthermore, the reduction in postoperative stiffness—one of the most problematic components of lesser toe deformity correction—makes it an attractive alternative to flexor-to-extensor transfer in many cases.

SUMMARY

Complex digital deformities and MTP joint instability encompass a wide range of pathologies, and we must identify the different degrees of ligamentous disruption. It is important to address a combination of procedures to treat gross deformities of the lesser toes that is, classified by an anatomic and clinical classification of lesser MTP joint instability.

Surgical treatment for these complex deformities should be individualized and requires a sequential process for adequate reduction and deformity correction. The FDL tendon transfer is just 1 option and typically just 1 part of a multitude of procedures that may include proximal interphalangeal joint arthrodesis, soft tissue rebalancing, other tendon transfers, and a metatarsal osteotomy. There is no one procedure that is the gold standard for every deformity. Although residual stiffness can result from the tendon transfer, overall patient satisfaction levels remain high when it is performed under the proper indications and concomitantly with other procedures to gain full correction of these challenging deformities.

REFERENCES

1. Nery C, Coughlin M, Baumfeld D, et al. How to classify plantar plate injuries: parameters from history and physical examination. Rev Bras Ortop 2015;50(6): 720–8.
2. Maas NM, van der Grinten M, Bramer WM, et al. Metatarsophalangeal joint stability: a systematic review on the plantar plate of the lesser toes. J Foot Ankle Res 2016;9:32.
3. Nery C, Umans H, Baumfeld D. Etiology, clinical assessment, and surgical repair of plantar plate tears. Semin Musculoskelet Radiol 2016;20(02): 205–13.
4. Suero EM, Meyers KN, Bohne WH. Stability of the metatarsophalangeal joint of the lesser toes: a cadaveric study. J Orthop Res 2012;30(12):1995–8.
5. Chalayon O, Chertman C, Guss AD, et al. Role of plantar plate and surgical reconstruction techniques on static stability of lesser metatarsophalangeal joints: a biomechanical study. Foot Ankle Int 2013;34(10):1436–42.
6. Barg A, Courville XF, Nickisch F, et al. Role of collateral ligaments in metatarsophalangeal stability: a cadaver study. Foot Ankle Int 2012;33(10):877–82.
7. Coughlin MJ, Baumfeld DS, Nery C. Second MTP joint instability: grading of the deformity and description of surgical repair of capsular insufficiency. Phys Sportsmed 2011;39(3):132–41.
8. Doty JF, Coughlin MJ. Metatarsophalangeal joint instability of the lesser toes. J Am Acad Orthop Surg 2014;22(4):235–45.
9. Nery C, Coughlin MJ, Baumfeld D, et al. Classification of metatarsophalangeal joint plantar plate injuries: history and physical examination variables. J Surg Orthop Adv 2014;23(4):214–23.
10. Hofstaetter SG, Hofstaetter JG, Petroutsas JA, et al. The Weil osteotomy: a seven-year follow-up. J Bone Joint Surg Br 2005;87(11):1507–11.
11. Baravarian B, Thompson J, Nazarian D. Plantar plate tears: a review of the modified flexor tendon transfer repair for stabilization. Clin Podiatric Med Surg 2011; 28(1):57–68.
12. Nery C, Coughlin MJ, Baumfeld D, et al. Lesser metatarsophalangeal joint instability: prospective evaluation and repair of plantar plate and capsular insufficiency. Foot Ankle Int 2012;33(4):301–11.

13. Klein EE, Weil L Jr, Weil LS Sr, et al. Positive drawer test combined with radiographic deviation of the third metatarsophalangeal joint suggests high grade tear of the second metatarsophalangeal joint plantar plate. Foot Ankle Spec 2014;7(6):466–70.

14. Nery C, Raduan FC, Catena F, et al. Plantar plate radiofrequency and Weil osteotomy for subtle metatarsophalangeal joint instability. J Orthop Surg Res 2015;10:180.

15. Barouk P, Barouk LS. Clinical diagnosis of gastrocnemius tightness. Foot Ankle Clin 2014;19(4):659–67.

16. Nery C, Coughlin MJ, Baumfeld D, et al. MRI evaluation of the MTP plantar plates compared with arthroscopic findings: a prospective study. Foot Ankle Int 2013; 34(3):315–22.

17. Umans R, Umans B, Umans H, et al. Predictive MRI Correlates of Lesser Metatarsophalangeal Joint (MPJ) Plantar Plate (PP) Tear. Radiological Society of North America 2014 Scientific Assembly and Annual Meeting. Chicago, IL, November 30-December 5, 2014.

18. Ford LA, Collins KB, Christensen JC. Stabilization of the subluxed second metatarsophalangeal joint: flexor tendon transfer versus primary repair of the plantar plate. J Foot Ankle Surg 1998;37(3):217–22.

19. Gazdag A, Cracchiolo A. Surgical treatment of patients with painful instability of the second metatarsophalangeal joint. Foot Ankle Int 1998;19(3): 137–43.

20. Cooper MT, Coughlin MJ. Sequential dissection for exposure of the second metatarsophalangeal joint. Foot Ankle Int 2011;32(3):294–9.

21. Veljkovic A, Lansang E, Lau J. Forefoot tendon transfers. Foot Ankle Clin 2014; 19(1):123–37.

22. Coughlin MJ, Schutt SA, Hirose CB, et al. Metatarsophalangeal joint pathology in crossover second toe deformity: a cadaveric study. Foot Ankle Int 2012;33(2): 133–40.

23. Butterworth M. Tendon transfers for management of digital and lesser metatarsophalangeal joint deformities. Clin Podiatr Med Surg 2016;33(1):71–84.

24. Becerro de Bengoa Vallejo R, Losa Iglesias ME, Prados Frutos JC, et al. Dorsal approach to transfer of the flexor digitorum brevis tendon. J Am Podiatr Med Assoc 2011;101(4):297–306.

25. Nery C, Coughlin MJ, Baumfeld D, et al. Prospective evaluation of protocol for surgical treatment of lesser MTP joint plantar plate tears. Foot Ankle Int 2014; 35(9):876–85.

26. Maestro M, Besse JL, Ragusa M, et al. Forefoot morphotype study and planning method for forefoot osteotomy. Foot Ankle Clin 2003;8(4):695–710.

27. Sorensen MD, Weil L Jr. Lesser metatarsal osteotomy. Clin Podiatric Med Surg 2015;32(3):275–90.

28. Dowd T, Bluman EM. Tendon transfers-how do they work? Foot Ankle Clin 2014; 19(1):17–27.

29. Thompson FM, Deland JT. Flexor tendon transfer for metatarsophalangeal instability of the second toe. Foot Ankle 1993;14(7):385–8.

30. Myers SH, Schon LC. Forefoot tendon transfers. Foot Ankle Clin 2011;16(3): 471–88.

31. Sung W. Technique using interference fixation repair for plantar plate ligament disruption of lesser metatarsophalangeal joints. J Foot Ankle Surg 2015;54(3): 508–12.

32. Kirchner JSMD, Wagner EMD. Girdlestone-Taylor flexor extensor tendon transfer. Tech Foot Ankle Surg 2004;3(2):91–9.

33. Haddad SL, Sabbagh RC, Resch S, et al. Results of flexor-to-extensor and extensor brevis tendon transfer for correction of the crossover second toe deformity. Foot Ankle Int 1999;20(12):781–8.

34. Becerro de Bengoa Vallejo R, Losa Iglesias ME, Rodriguez MF, et al. Single longitudinal dorsal incision approach to transfer the flexor digitorum longus tendon between the flexor digitorum brevis hemitendons: a cadaveric study. J Am Podiatr Med Assoc 2013;103(5):430–7.

35. Rippstein PF, Park YU. A modified technique for flexor-to-extensor tendon transfer to correct residual metatarsophalangeal extension in the treatment of hammertoes. J Foot Ankle Surg 2014;53(6):810–2.

36. Shurnas PSMD, Sanders APAC. Second MTP joint capsular instability with clawing deformity: metatarsal osteotomy, flexor transfer with biotenodesis, hammer toe repair, and MTP arthroplasty without the need for plantar incisions. Tech Foot Ankle Surg 2005;4(3):196–201.

37. DiPaolo ZJ, Ross MS, Laughlin RT, et al. Proximal phalanx and flexor digitorum longus tendon biomechanics in flexor to extensor tendon transfer. Foot Ankle Int 2015;36(5):585–90.

38. Haddad SLMD. The crossover toe: use of extensor tendons in transfer techniques. Tech Foot Ankle Surg 2008;7(1):45–51.

39. Barca F, Acciaro AL. Surgical correction of crossover deformity of the second toe: a technique for tenodesis. Foot Ankle Int 2004;25(9):620–4.

40. Lui TH, Chan KB. Technique tip: modified extensor digitorum brevis tendon transfer for crossover second toe correction. Foot Ankle Int 2007;28(4):521–3.

41. Hobizal KB, Wukich DK, Manway J. Extensor digitorum brevis transfer technique to correct multiplanar deformity of the lesser digits. Foot Ankle Specialist 2016; 9(3):252–7.

42. Myerson MS, Jung HG. The role of toe flexor-to-extensor transfer in correcting metatarsophalangeal joint instability of the second toe. Foot Ankle Int 2005; 26(9):675–9.

43. Nery CMD, Baumfeld DMD. Salvage of lesser toes deformities: "revision forefoot". Tech Foot Ankle Surg 2017;16(1):20–7.

44. Peck CN, Macleod A, Barrie J. Lesser metatarsophalangeal instability: presentation, management, and outcomes. Foot Ankle Int 2012;33(7):565–70.

45. Good J, Fiala K. Digital surgery: current trends and techniques. Clin Podiatric Med Surg 2010;27(4):583–99.

46. Losa Iglesias ME, Becerro de Bengoa Vallejo R, Jules KT, et al. Meta-analysis of flexor tendon transfer for the correction of lesser toe deformities. J Am Podiatr Med Assoc 2012;102(5):359–68.

47. Highlander P, VonHerbulis E, Gonzalez A, et al. Complications of the Weil osteotomy. Foot Ankle Spec 2011;4(3):165–70.

48. Mendicino RW, Statler TK, Saltrick KR, et al. Predislocation syndrome: a review and retrospective analysis of eight patients. J Foot Ankle Surg 2001;40(4): 214–24.

APPENDIX 1: COMBINATION OF CLINICAL AND ANATOMIC GRADING SYSTEMS FOR LESSER TOES PLANTAR PLATE TEARS WAS POSSIBLE BECAUSE OF THE HIGH CORRELATION FOUND BETWEEN THE CLINICAL FINDINGS AND ANATOMIC TYPES OF TEARS.

Grade	Alignment	Physical Examination	Surgical Anatomy
Zero	MTPJ aligned Prodromal phase No deformity	MTPJ pain MTPJ swelling Reduced Toe Purchase Negative MTPJ Drawer	Attenuation
One	MTPJ mild malalignment Widening web space Toe Medial Deviation	MTPJ pain Mild swelling Loss of Toe Purchase Mild MTPJ Drawer <50 % = subluxable	Partial Transverse Distal Tear
Two	MTPJ moderate malalignment Medial, lateral or dorsal deformity Hyperextension of the toe	MTPJ pain Reduced swelling No Toe Purchase Moderate MTPJ Drawer >50 % = subluxable	Complete Transverse Distal Tear
Three	MTPJ severe malalignment Dorsomedial deformity (cross-over toe) Flexible Hammertoe	MTPJ and toe pain Reduced swelling No Toe Purchase Very positive MTPJ Drawer (Dislocatable MTPJ) Flexible Hammertoe	Combination of Transverse and Longitudinal Tears
Four	MTPJ severe deformity Dorsomedial or dorsal dislocation Fixed Hammertoe	MTPJ and toe pain Little or no swelling No Toe Purchase Dislocated MTPJ Fixed Hammertoe	Extensive Tear with button-hole

Reprinted from the Southern Orthopaedic Association Nery C, Coughlin MJ, Baumfeld D, et al. Classification of metatarsophalangeal joint plantar plate injuries: history and physical examination variables. J Surg Orthop Adv 2014;23(4):214–23; with permission.

Lesser Metatarsophalangeal Joint Instability
Advancements in Plantar Plate Reconstruction

Raymond Y. Hsu, MD*, Alexej Barg, MD, Florian Nickisch, MD

KEYWORDS

- Plantar plate • Collateral ligaments • Lesser metatarsophalangeal joint
- Lesser metatarsophalangeal joint instability • Plantar plate repair

KEY POINTS

- The plantar plate and collateral ligaments are the primary stabilizers of the lesser metatarsophalangeal joints.
- Clinical history and examination is very reliable for diagnosing plantar plate pathology.
- Beyond plain radiographs, MRI should be reserved for ambiguous cases, and arthrogram with fluoroscopy and concomitant corticosteroid injection can be both diagnostic and therapeutic.
- The dorsal approach avoids a plantar scar and permits substantial flexibility with additional procedures including extensor tendon lengthening, Weil osteotomy, hammertoe correction, and a flexor-to-extensor transfer if the plantar plate is irreparable.
- The clinical results of a dorsal approach to plantar plate repairs are promising with respect to pain relief and patient satisfaction.

INTRODUCTION

Plantar plate tears have been established as an underlying pathology for a range of lesser metatarsophalangeal (MTP) conditions including synovitis, metatarsalgia, instability, frank dislocation, crossover toe, and interphalangeal toe pathology, such as hammertoe and claw toe.[1–3] Anatomic and biomechanical studies have demonstrated the plantar plate and collateral ligaments to be the primary stabilizers of the lesser MTP joints.[4–8] Lesser MTP pathology that may have been previously treated with some combination of extensor tendon lengthening, MTP soft tissue release, Weil

Disclosures: Dr F. Nickisch receives royalties from Smith and Nephew for the Hat-Trick Lesser Toe Repair System. Drs R.Y. Hsu and A. Barg have nothing to disclose.
Department of Orthopedics, The University of Utah, 590 Wakara Way, Salt Lake City, UT 84108, USA
* Corresponding author.
E-mail address: raymond_hsu@brown.edu

Foot Ankle Clin N Am 23 (2018) 127–143
https://doi.org/10.1016/j.fcl.2017.09.009
1083-7515/18/© 2017 Elsevier Inc. All rights reserved.

foot.theclinics.com

osteotomy, flexor-to-extensor transfer, and K-wire transfixion, and may now be treated more anatomically by incorporating a plantar plate repair.[1,2] As clinical experience with plantar plate repair grows, the indications, role, and outcomes are becoming better defined.[9–12]

ANATOMY AND BIOMECHANICS
Plantar Plate

The normal anatomy of the plantar plate has been well-characterized in cadaveric studies (**Fig. 1**).[4,5] The normal plantar plate is a flexible but inelastic structure on average 19 mm in length and 2 mm thick.[4,5] It is trapezoidal in shape with an average width proximally of 11 mm at its metatarsal attachment and 9 mm at its proximal phalangeal attachment.[5] The dorsal aspect of the normal plantar plate is described as "articular appearing," essentially an extension of the concave articular surface of the proximal phalanx, cupping the metatarsal head.[4] The plantar aspect of the plantar plate is centrally grooved, forming the dorsal aspect of the flexor tendon sheaths (**Fig. 2**).[4,5] Correspondingly, the medial and lateral aspects of the plantar plate are thicker than the central portion.[4,5]

Distally, the plantar plate has a firm fibrous attachment directly into the proximal phalanx immediately adjacent to the articular surface (**Fig. 3**).[4,5,13] Proximally, the direct attachment to the metatarsal just proximal to the articular surface has the appearance of thin connective tissue grossly and synovial tissue histologically.[4,5] Based on appearance alone, the mechanical contribution of this direct proximal attachment may be negligible. The accessory collateral ligaments provide a stouter indirect connection between the metatarsal and the plantar plate, creating a sling that supports the metatarsal head.[4,5] The other proximal mechanically relevant connections are primarily from other soft tissue structures. The plantar fascia terminates on stout insertions into the proximal plantar plate.[4] The deep transverse metatarsal ligaments span across adjacent plantar plates confluent with the plantar fibers of the proximal two-thirds of each plate, providing even more proximal restraint.[4,5,14] The lumbricals and interossei insert on the proximal phalanx, but also have fibers inserting into the distal plantar plate.[4,5]

Histologically, the plantar plate is fibrocartilage with the majority of fibers running longitudinally with some interwoven oblique fibers.[4,5] The collagen is 75% type 1 and there is minimal to no elastin.[4,5] Proximally, in the plantar one-third, fibers are positioned transversely, continuous with the deep transverse metatarsal ligament.[4]

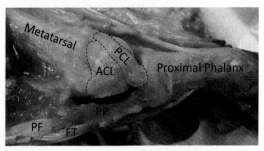

Fig. 1. Medial dissection of a lesser metatarsophalangeal joint with the proper collateral ligament (PCL) released from the proximal phalanx and accessory collateral ligament (ACL) released from the plantar plate (PP). The attachment of the distal plantar fascia (PF) to the PP and relative position of the flexor tendons (FT) is also demonstrated.

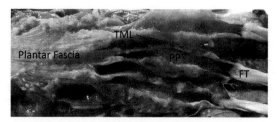

Fig. 2. Plantar dissection of the foot with the flexor tendon sheaths opened and the flexor tendons (FT) cut proximally and reflected distally. The major proximal attachments to the plantar plate (PP) are demonstrated: the plantar fascia and the deep transverse metatarsal ligament (TML).

Histologic preparations of the distal plantar plate confirm that it interdigitates into the subchondral bone of the phalanx and the dorsal plantar plate is confluent with the hyaline cartilage of the phalanx.[13]

The functions of the plantar plate as derived from its anatomy can be divided into at least 2 categories: weight bearing and joint stability. Its fibrocartilage structure, similar to that of the meniscus of the knee or the annulus fibrosus of the spine, dictates a weight bearing role cushioning and dissipating ground forces to the metatarsal head.[4,5] Anecdotally, this anomaly is reflected in the patient complaint of "walking on marbles" when the plantar plate is torn.[2] Its direct stout attachment to the proximal phalanx distally, its multiple fibrous restraints proximally, and its predominantly longitudinal fibers reflect its role stabilizing the MTP joint.[4,5]

Collateral Ligaments

The MTP collateral ligaments, although anatomically and functionally integrated with the plantar plate, warrant specific discussion. As a layer, the collateral ligaments are confluent with the dorsal capsule, but are discrete structures arising from the metatarsal tubercles high and proximal along the medial and lateral aspects of the

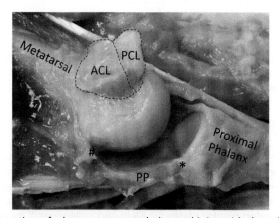

Fig. 3. Medial dissection of a lesser metatarsophalangeal joint with the collateral ligaments (accessory collateral ligament [ACL] and proper collateral ligament [PCL]) released distally and reflected proximally on their origins. Traction demonstrates the stout distal attachment (*asterisk*) of the plantar plate (PP) confluent with the phalanx articular surface. The proximal attachment (*hash*) to the metatarsal is thin and synovial.

metatarsal head.[4,5] From each metatarsal tubercle, the collateral ligament fans out in a plantar direction as 2 components as it progresses distally. The more dorsal proper collateral ligament component attaches directly on the plantar most aspect of the side of the proximal phalanx.[4] The more plantar accessory collateral ligament component inserts more broadly along the entire side of the plantar plate.[4] This is the major attachment of the plantar plate to the metatarsal, anatomically demonstrating the contribution of the collateral ligament to not only coronal but also sagittal plane stability.

Mechanics: Plantar Plate and Collateral Ligaments

Biomechanical cadaveric studies have repeatedly confirmed the crucial role of the plantar plate and the collateral ligaments in the stability of the lesser MTP joint. Bhatia and colleagues[6] demonstrated that isolated sectioning of either the plantar plate or the collateral ligaments permits the MTP joint to completely dorsally dislocate with forces that would otherwise not even cause 2.5 mm of dorsal displacement. Furthermore, combined compromise of both the plantar plate and the collateral ligaments permitted dislocation at even lower forces.[6] Chalayon and colleagues[7] expanded on these findings and demonstrated that the plantar plate resists not only dorsal subluxation, but also stabilizes MTP dorsiflexion and plantarflexion. Wang and colleagues[14] further showed that even cutting the deep transverse metatarsal ligaments that connect adjacent plantar plates was sufficient to introduce instability, and decreased resistance against dorsiflexion and plantarflexion and dorsal subluxation.

The specific contribution of the collateral ligaments to MTP sagittal stability in the setting of intact plantar plates has also been investigated. Deland and colleagues[15] demonstrated that with transection of the dorsal capsule and both collateral ligaments in cadaveric lesser MTP joints, the previously stable joints grossly dorsally dislocated on repeat manual stress examination. Barg and colleagues[8] investigated the mechanical effect of transecting only the lateral collateral ligament in cadaveric specimens, keeping the medial ligament and plantar plate intact. Even unilateral collateral ligament compromise caused a decrease in stiffness with respect to dorsal translation. Isolated release of the accessory collateral ligament, which inserts on the plantar plate introduced more dorsal instability than isolated release of the proper collateral ligament, which inserts on the proximal phalanx.[8]

In summary, these mechanical cadaveric studies have reinforced the findings from previous anatomic studies establishing the plantar plate and collateral ligaments as the primary sagittal stabilizers of the lesser MTP joints.[4–8,15] The specific numerical findings of each mechanical study are not reported here because there is too much variability in experimental protocols to allow for meaningful cross-study comparisons.[6–8,15]

CLINICAL EVALUATION
Presentation and Examination

Pain is generally the presenting symptom with concomitant deformity if there is substantial loss of dorsal restraint, involvement of unilateral collateral ligaments, or asymmetric involvement of the plantar plate.[2,16,17] Plantar plate tears can occur after an acute injury or present as chronic attritional metatarsalgia. A retrospective series of 100 operatively treated plantar plates by Klein and colleagues[16] found that 7% presented with sudden onset of pain and 93% presented with gradual onset. Similarly, in a series of 28 patients by Nery and colleagues,[17] 10% attributed their symptoms to an acute injury. Patients may complain of "walking on marbles," especially with barefoot ambulation on hard surfaces or with uncushioned shoe wear.

An antalgic gait may be apparent as the patient tries to offload the affected joint. If acutely inflamed, swelling and dorsal tenderness over the MTP joint are common. Plantar tenderness at the metatarsal head raises suspicion of loss of cushioning of the plantar plate.[2] Klein and colleagues[16] found in their series of operatively treated plantar plates that plantar pain and edema at the second metatarsal head had a high incidence (98% for pain and 92% for edema) and sensitivity (98% for pain and 85.8% for edema), but were nonspecific (11.1% for both). The nonmechanical signs and symptoms described are all nonspecific and may also be attributed to other causes of metatarsalgia, including overload, synovitis, focal chondral injuries, arthritis, capsular injuries, stress fractures, and neuromas.

Signs or symptoms of the loss of mechanical stability of a plantar plate injury are diagnostically more specific. A hammertoe or crossover toe or simply a dorsiflexed position of the proximal phalanx raises suspicion of an incompetent plantar plate.[2,3,16] The stability of the MTP joint can also be directly assessed by a vertical stress or drawer test as described by Thompson and Hamilton (**Fig. 4**).[1] Klein and colleagues[16] found the drawer test to be the most specific (99.8%) clinical examination finding.[1] The MTP joint is held in neutral or slightly dorsiflexed position and then a vertical shear force is placed on the proximal phalanx to displace it dorsally.[1,15] The degree of translation and any elicited pain is noted.[1] Comparison with the adjacent and contralateral toes is useful.[18]

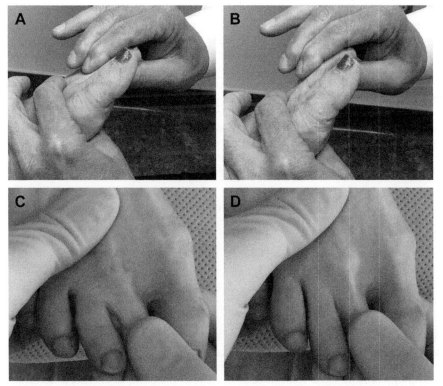

Fig. 4. Drawer test demonstrated from side view (*A, B*) and from examiner's view (*C, D*). The distal metatarsal and proximal phalanx are stabilized independently (*A, C*). With dorsal stress applied (*B, D*), instability is assessed.

Imaging: Radiographs

Weight bearing anteroposterior, lateral, and oblique radiographs of the foot should be routine in the workup of lesser MTP pain. Radiographs may increase suspicion of a plantar plate or collateral ligament injury if there is dorsal subluxation or medial/lateral deviation, respectively, of the proximal phalanx on the metatarsal head. Subtle cases may benefit from comparison with contralateral radiographs. In more severe cases, radiographs may confirm complete dislocation of the lesser MTP joint, which is anatomically impossible without compromise of the plantar plate. Aside from the alignment of the MTP joint, radiographs may be diagnostic of other conditions in the differential including stress fractures, Freiberg's disease, degenerative arthrosis, or systemic arthritis.[1,19] The full set of 3 views of the foot instead of dedicated toe radiographs also allows the identification of any proximal pathology or architecture, such as a longer metatarsal, that may be driving the forefoot pain.

Imaging: MRI

With the high accuracy of clinical examination for diagnosing plantar plate tears, MRI is most appropriately reserved for cases when the diagnosis and treatment plan cannot be established from the clinical findings.[11,16,20] The normal plantar plate appears on MRI as a low-signal smooth structure following the contour of the metatarsal head and inserting on the proximal phalanx (**Fig. 5**).[13,18,21] The plantar plate must be carefully distinguished from the also hypointense flexor tendons immediately plantar, because there is often no discrete interval.[18,21] On T2-weighted sequences, the distal insertional fibers of the normal plantar plate may be mildly hyperintense and the higher signal articular cartilage of the phalanx undercuts the insertion of the normal plantar plate. These normal focally hyperintense patterns can be confused for the true pathology of a plantar plate tear, which also usually appears as hyperintense signal near the distal attachment (**Figs. 6** and **7**).[13,18,21] To differentiate, the signal change of a plantar plate tear is typically higher in intensity and extends proximally from the distal attachment over a greater distance, representing a true discontinuity.[19–22] The region of rupture is nearly isointense with the synovium and synovial fluid.[21,22] Other associated signs on MRI include joint effusion, fluid in the flexor tendon sheath, and synovitis.[20–22]

The accuracy of MRI in diagnosing plantar plate tears has been assessed in multiple studies using intraoperative findings as the reference standard.[18,20,23] Sung and

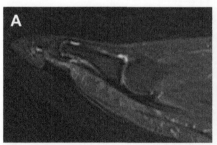 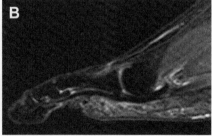

Fig. 5. Example MRI images of 2 asymptomatic second MTP joints demonstrating how normal plantar plates can be misinterpreted as torn. (*A*) Sagittal T2-weighted MRI demonstrating hyperintense signal from articular cartilage of the proximal phalanx undercutting the attachment of the plantar plate, which can be confused with a tear. (*B*) Sagittal short T1 inversion recovery MRI demonstrating normal distal fibers of the plantar plate that may also be hyperintense.

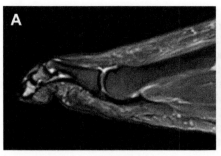
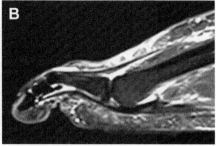

Fig. 6. (*A*) Sagittal T2-weighted MRI of a second MTP with metatarsalgia with normal appearing plantar plate. (*B*) Sagittal short T1 inversion recovery MRI of the same second MTP 2 years later with diffuse increased signal in the distal plantar plate indicative of a tear.

colleagues[20] looked at the preoperative MRIs of 45 second MTP joints. There were 39 plantar plate tears diagnosed on MRI, all of which were confirmed intraoperatively. Of the 6 plantar plates diagnosed as intact on MRI, 2 were also found to be torn intraoperatively. Overall, Sung and colleagues[20] found preoperative MRI to have a sensitivity of 95% and specificity of 100%. Klein and colleagues[23] with the same senior authors repeated this study with 51 second MTP joints, 46 of which had tears found intraoperatively, and found MRI to have a sensitivity of 74% and specificity of 100%. Both studies had an experienced musculoskeletal radiologist reading the MRIs and paying particular attention to different plantar plate tear patterns and grades.[17]

A separate group, Nery and colleagues[18] compared MRIs with intraoperative arthroscopy of 55 symptomatic second, third, and fourth MTP joints. They similarly found that, with an experienced radiologist paying particular attention to different plantar plate tear patterns, the sensitivity and specificity of MRI was high, at 96% and 81%, respectively.[17,18] The sensitivity of MRI was significantly lower, at 14% to 36%, when read by either resident radiologists or radiologists unfamiliar with plantar plate tear patterns.[18]

With respect to pretest probability, the 3 studies discussed were all done in patient populations where the clinical suspicion of a plantar plate tear was already sufficiently high to proceed with an MRI and to surgery.[18,20,23] Gregg and colleagues[24] evaluated

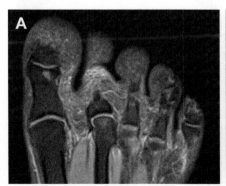
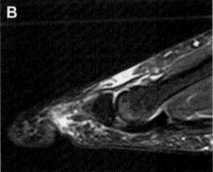

Fig. 7. (*A*) Axial proton density MRI of a forefoot with second metatarsophalangeal (MTP) metatarsalgia and instability demonstrating a second MTP lateral collateral ligament tear. (*B*) Sagittal short T1 inversion recovery MRI of the same second MTP showing bony edema and distal plantar plate diffuse increased signal consistent with a plantar plate tear.

all the lesser MTP joints in 40 symptomatic forefeet (160 MTP joints), of which only 10 feet (25 MTP joints) underwent surgical correction as dictated by clinical findings, and MRI diagnosed tears in 89% of the plantar plates. Furthermore, in a comparative group of 40 asymptomatic feet, MRI diagnosed tears in 35% of the plantar plates.[24] The high rate of MRI diagnosis of plantar plate tears in toes adjacent to symptomatic toes and in completely asymptomatic feet supports cautious interpretation when MTP joints are not symptomatic. As with most MRI examinations, use should be judicious for the diagnosis of plantar plate tears and interpretation should be performed in the clinical context. In most cases, clinical examination is sufficient to dictate the diagnosis and treatment, and MRI is not indicated.[11]

Imaging: Arthrography

Arthrography with fluoroscopy structurally tests the integrity of the plantar plate but also the MTP joint capsule in general.[25–27] A 25-G needle is used to inject radiopaque contrast directly into the MTP joint. Extension of the contrast into the flexor tendon sheath is diagnostic for a plantar plate rupture (**Fig. 8**).[22,25–27] Additional patterns of

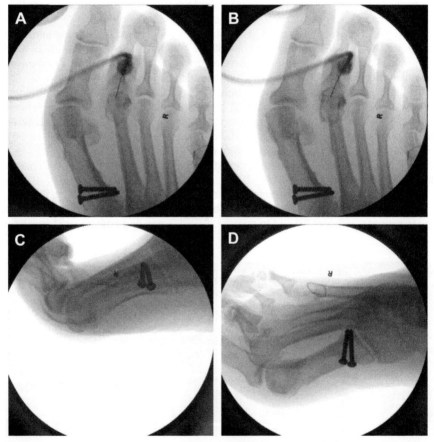

Fig. 8. Fluoroscopically guided injection into a second metatarsophalangeal joint. The arthrogram initially seems to be normal (*A*), but the contrast subsequently extravasates proximally (*B*). Additional images (*C, D*) confirm that the contrast is in the flexor tendon sheath, indicative of a plantar plate tear.

extravasation have also been identified that are indicative of collateral ligament or joint capsule tears (**Fig. 9**).[25,27] Mazzuca and colleagues[27] used arthrography with fluoroscopy to evaluate the integrity of the plantar plates and joint capsules of 40 lesser MTP joints. Using MRI arthrography as the reference, they found plain arthrography to have a sensitivity of 88% and a specificity of 63%.[27] Of the 25 toes with available intraoperative findings for reference, plain arthrography again demonstrated a sensitivity of 88% and no cases with normal arthrograms proceeded to surgery to calculate a meaningful specificity.[27] They also noted during the course of their study that adding additional oblique fluoroscopic views improved the accuracy of plain arthrography to be equivalent to MRI arthrography.[27]

Arthrography with fluoroscopy is an attractive adjunct in the management of painful lesser MTP instability. Beyond the diagnostic ability of the imaging, concurrent injection of lidocaine or other local anesthetic into the joint can confirm an intraarticular pain generator. The addition of a corticosteroid may provide temporary or lasting relief and potentially avoid a surgical intervention.[28–30] It is also more affordable than MRI.[27] Especially when treating a painful lesser MTP without deformity, a corticosteroid injection along with shoe wear modifications and metatarsal pads should be trialed before considering operative intervention.[2,19,28–30]

SURGICAL TREATMENT AND OUTCOMES
Plantar Plate Repair: Plantar Approach

Although the plantar approach to the plantar plate has been repeatedly described and intuitively would be more direct, there are limited clinical reports.[2,25,31,32] Powless and Elze[25] reported a series of 58 MTP capsular repairs, of which only a minority were lesser plantar plate tears, and even fewer were repaired primarily through a plantar approach. They found that, even when repaired through a plantar approach, a dorsal accessory approach was often necessary to localize the tear from the inside out. Of the 15 patients who were available at mean follow-up of 30 months, all reported complete pain relief but fewer than one-half had undergone a plantar plate repair.[25]

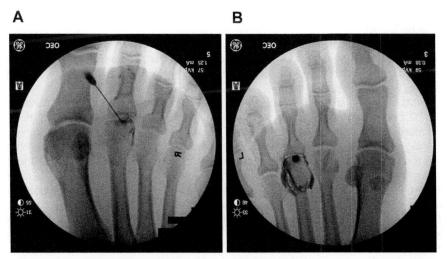

Fig. 9. Examples of additional patterns of extravasation: distal along the tendon sheath (*A*) and lateral through the lateral capsule or collateral ligament (*B*).

Bouché and Heit[31] reported on 17 feet in 15 patients with mean follow-up of 37 months; however, all had flexor-to-extensor tendon transfers along with the plantar plate repairs.

More recently, Prissel and colleagues[32] published a retrospective series of 144 lesser plantar plate repairs in 131 patients through a plantar approach without tendon transfers. Complications included 6 wound problems (4.2%), 11 recurrences (7.6%), and 4 revisions (2.8%). Surveys were completed by 72 patients representing 76 repairs at mean follow-up of 22 months. The mean visual analog scale (VAS) score was 2.3, but 31.6% attributed their pain to the plantar scar. With respect to patient satisfaction, 55.3% were satisfied with the procedure and would have the surgery again.[32]

Plantar Plate Repair: Dorsal Approach

The dorsal approach to the plantar plate has gained traction because it avoids potentially painful plantar scars and a single incision can access adjacent MTP joints as well as be extended to address interphalangeal pathology.[9–12,17,33–36] Cooper and Coughlin in a small cadaveric study showed that with (1) dorsal extensor tendon release, (2) capsulotomy, and (3) the release of the collaterals distally off the proximal phalanx, approximately 5 mm of the plantar plate can be visualized.[33] The addition of a Weil osteotomy allowed visualization of 8 mm of the plantar plate.[33] They, along with other authors, concluded that, without a Weil osteotomy, dorsal exposure is not sufficient for a safe plantar plate repair.[33,35]

Jastifer and Coughlin, however, in a subsequent cadaver study demonstrated that with (1) dorsal capsulotomy, (2) release of the collaterals off the metatarsal head, (3) passing a McGlamry elevator to release the proximal synovial attachments, and (4) release of the plantar plate off the proximal phalanx, a mean exposure of 5.3 mm and minimum of 4.3 mm was achieved.[34] More technically relevant was the demonstration that, even without a Weil osteotomy, 2 sutures were successfully passed through the plantar plate with the use of a commercially available suture passer in all 12 specimens.[34] Nonetheless, to date, the majority of published clinical experience with plantar plate repair through a dorsal approach incorporates a Weil osteotomy, whether for exposure or owing to the continued belief that shortening the affected ray is beneficial.[9–12,17]

The authors of published case series to date also consistently advocate for first trialing conservative measures before considering plantar pate repair.[9–12] All series excluded patients with neurologic disorders or rheumatoid arthritis.[9–12] Most excluded patients with diabetes mellitus.[9,11,12]

Gregg and colleagues[12] published the first retrospective series of a single surgeon with 35 dorsal approach plantar plate repairs with Weil osteotomies (second, third, and fourth MTPs) in 23 feet in 21 patients. The mean follow-up was 26 months (range, 19–36). Four of the patients were only able to follow up by phone, but of the 17 patients who followed up clinically, 1 had a marked recurrent dorsal subluxation and the 2 others had mildly increased sagittal extension. Preoperatively, pain was severe in 15 feet, moderate in 6, and mild in 2. Postoperatively, 1 was moderately painful, 4 were mildly painful, and 18 were pain free. With respect to activity, postoperatively, 10 feet were noted to cause intermittent or occasional limitations and 13 caused no limitation. Complications included 4 cases of infection treated with local wound care and oral antibiotics, 2 cases of painful hardware treated with removal of hardware, and 1 case of transfer metatarsalgia. Of the 23 feet, the patients were dissatisfied with 6 (26%) and satisfied with 17 (74%).[12]

Weil and colleagues[10] published his retrospective series of 15 dorsal approach second MTP plantar plate repairs with Weil osteotomies in 13 patients. The mean follow-up was 22.5 months (range, 13–32). The mean VAS improved from 7.3 preoperatively to 1.7 postoperatively ($P<.0001$). There were no cases of recurrent instability. Complications included 1 case of metatarsalgia and 3 cases of painful hardware, with 1 removal of hardware. Of the 15 repairs, the patients were dissatisfied with 3 (20%) and satisfied with 12 (80%).[10]

Nery and colleagues[17] prospectively enrolled his patients and published their experience of 40 dorsal approach lesser MTP plantar plate repairs in 22 patients. This series was then expanded and included in a larger series of 100 MTP plantar plate treatments in 68 patients.[9] Unique to this series, all MTP joints first underwent arthroscopy to grade the plantar tears according to Coughlin and colleagues[3] and undergo a synovectomy as indicated. The grade of the tear then dictated the treatment, all of which included a Weil osteotomy.[9] Grade 0 (plantar plate attenuation) and grade I (transverse distal or midsubstance tears of <50%) were treated with radiofrequency shrinkage. Grade II (transverse distal or midsubstance tears of >50%) and grade III (transverse tears and/or longitudinal extensive tears) were treated with dorsal approach direct repair. Grade IV (extensive tears with button hole or extensive combination transverse and longitudinal tears), were treated with a flexor-to-extensor tendon transfer.

For all 100 plantar plate tears in the series from Nery and colleagues,[9] the mean follow-up was 24 months (range, 12–48). There were a total of 48 grade II and grade III tears treated with dorsal approach plantar plate repair. For the grade II tears, the mean VAS improved from 7.8 to 0.7 ($P<.0001$). For the grade III tears, the mean VAS improved from 8 to 1.2 ($P<.0001$). With respect to mean American Orthopaedic Foot and Ankle Society scores, the grade II tears improved from 48.3 preoperatively to 88.9 postoperatively ($P<.001$) and the grade III tears improved from 42.4 to 84.7 ($P<.001$). Complications and patient satisfaction were not reported.[9,17]

Most recently, in the largest series to date, Flint and colleagues[11] reported on the results of 2 senior surgeons with 138 dorsal approach plantar plate repairs in 97 feet in 91 patients. All but 2 of the plantar plate repairs incorporated a Weil osteotomy and follow-up results were all reported at 12 months. Only 15 plantar plate repairs were isolated. As with other published series, the vast majority of toes underwent concomitant procedures, the most common being interphalangeal corrections, hallux valgus procedures, and hallux MTP fusions. The mean VAS improved from 5.4 to 1.5 ($P<.001$). The mean American Orthopaedic Foot and Ankle Society score improved from 49 to 81 ($P<.001$). Before surgery, all 138 MTP joints had positive drawer examinations, ranging from less than 50% subluxation with stress to persistent dislocation without stress. At the final follow-up, only 6 had a positive drawer examination, none worse than less than 50% subluxation with stress. For the 97 feet, patients reported poor satisfaction scores for 4 (4.1%), fair for 15 (15.5%), and good to excellent for 78 (80.4%). For the 11 feet in the subset of 15 isolated plantar plate repairs, patients reported good to excellent satisfaction scores in 100%, but the study was not powered to compare between subsets of patients.[11]

There was a significant loss of both active and passive range of motion after repair, although the authors note that this is inherent to a stability procedure.[11] There were only 2 grade IV tears treated in the series reported by Flint and colleagues,[11] and the authors agree that with these tears with inadequate tissue, a flexor-to-extensor transfer is the treatment of choice.[9] No complications were reported in the 138 repairs included in the series, but there were 3 plantar plate repairs during the study period that did not resolve symptoms and underwent revision MTP procedures.[11] A fourth repair developed transfer metatarsalgia and a hammertoe in an adjacent toe, which then also underwent operative treatment. These 4 cases were excluded owing to not meeting follow-up requirements.[11]

Authors' Preferred Technique

Our preferred surgical technique for plantar plate repair is through a dorsal approach similar to what has been described (**Fig. 10**).[2,10,35] The dorsal approach eliminates plantar scarring and allows a single incision to address adjacent MTPs, lengthen or

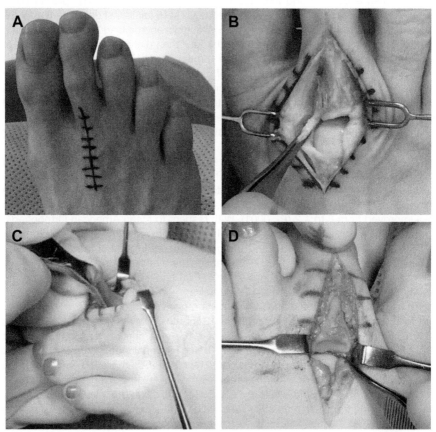

Fig. 10. Technique. (*A*) Dorsal incision over the lesser metatarsophalangeal (MTP) joint. (*B*) After mobilization of the extensor tendons, a longitudinal capsulotomy is made and the capsule is elevated taking care to preserve the collateral ligament origins proximally. (*C*) The plantar plate and collateral ligaments are release distally and a McGlamry elevator is used to mobilize the plantar plate proximally. (*D*) The toe is flexed to prepare the footprint of the plantar plate and collaterals on the proximal phalanx with a rasp or rongeur. (*E*) A suture passer is used to place 2 sutures in the plantar plate and 1 in the plantar aspect of each collateral ligament. (*F*) Two oblique nonintersecting drill holes are made with 1.6-mm K-wires through drill guides exiting plantar medially and laterally on the proximal phalanx. (*G*) After passing all 4 plantar plate and collateral ligament sutures through the drill holes, provisional tensioning is performed with the MTP joint reduced and slightly flexed. (*H*) Once the MTP is determined to be stable, the sutures are tied over the dorsal bone bridge. If interference wires are used, they are cut or removed at this time.

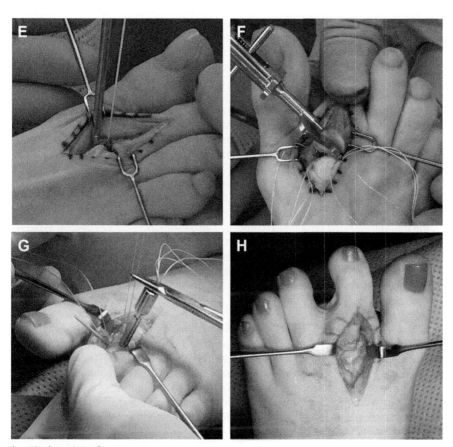

Fig. 10. (*continued*).

transfer extensor tendons, perform a Weil osteotomy, and address any interphalangeal deformity as indicated. We agree with some previous authors that history and examination in most cases are sufficient to confidently diagnose and direct treatment.[11,16] In our experience, MRI is useful only if the diagnosis is truly in question. We do find an arthrogram with fluoroscopy to be useful in confirming the diagnosis but predominantly to confirm an intraarticular pain generator and concomitantly deliver a corticosteroid injection. All patients should have exhausted conservative measures with shoe modifications, inserts with padding, metatarsal pads, and possibly a corticosteroid injection before considering an operative treatment. Patients are also made aware that if the plantar plate is irreparable owing to insufficient tissue, a flexor-to-extensor transfer is possible.[9,11]

1. *Incision*: A dorsal incision is made over the affected lesser MTP joint. If 2 adjacent MTPs are to be addressed or if a lateral release is to be performed for a hallux valgus correction, the incision is shifted to between MTP joints.
2. *Extensor tendons*: If there is an extension contracture of the MTP joint, the extensor tendons are transected to allow for Z-lengthening or a brevis to longus transfer. If there is no contracture, the extensor tendons are simply mobilized to expose the dorsal capsule.

3. *Dorsal capsule*: A longitudinal capsulotomy is made and elevated as 1 layer off the metatarsal dorsally and the phalanx dorsally, medially, and laterally. Care is taken to preserve the metatarsal origins of the collateral ligaments. Manual traction is applied to visualize the plantar plate and confirm the tear with a Freer elevator or small probe.

4. *Plantar plate and collateral release*: The collateral ligaments are sharply released from the proximal phalanx. The synovial attachments of the plantar plate on the plantar metatarsal are released with a McGlamry elevator. Whatever plantar plate remains attached to the phalanx is then released as well. The phalanx is plantar-flexed to allow preparation of the phalangeal footprint of the plantar plate and collaterals with a rasp.

5. *Weil osteotomy*: We only perform a Weil osteotomy if the second metatarsal is relatively longer on radiographs and/or there is a prominent plantar callous. If performed, we resect a thin wafer to prevent plantar translation and temporarily pin the metatarsal head proximally to improve visualization.[9,12,35] We believe avoiding a Weil osteotomy decreases the risk of a floating toe.

6. *Visualization*: In many cases, even without a Weil osteotomy, manual distraction of the toe is sufficient to visualize the plantar plate.[11,34] If not, a small pin-based distractor is placed dorsally spanning the MTP joint to assist in visualization.

7. *Passing plantar plate sutures:* Passing a suture through the plantar plate simply with a small atraumatic curved needle has been well-described, although always with a Weil osteotomy.[12,17,36] We believe that, without the osteotomy, better purchase of the plantar plate can be more safely obtained with a dedicated suture passer such as from the Viper (Arthrex, Naples, FL) or Hat-Trick (Smith and Nephew, London, UK) systems.[34] Two 2-0 nonabsorbable sutures are passed as simple cinch stitches, one for each side (medial and lateral) of the plantar plate. The sutures are tested gently to confirm that there is adequate purchase. If the plantar plate tissue is too poor to hold sutures, a flexor to extensor transfer is performed instead.

8. *Passing collateral ligament sutures:* Two 2-0 nonabsorbable sutures of a different color are also passed as cinch stitches to capture each collateral ligament proximally. Care is taken to ensure that the sutures are passed sufficiently plantar through the collaterals in the stouter tissue. We have also found that passing the collateral sutures too dorsally sets the joint up for a floating toe deformity. Reefing the collaterals after the plantar plate repair has been described.[9,11,35] We believe, however, that passing dedicated sutures in the plantar aspect of the collaterals for eventual attachment to the plantar phalanx more anatomically replicates the native oblique orientation of the accessory collateral ligament/ proper collateral ligament and may decrease the risk of a floating toe.

9. *Proximal phalanx drill holes*: A 1.6-mm K-wire is used to prepare 2 drill holes in the proximal phalanx. Drilling obliquely from the dorsal to plantar allows the tunnels to exit plantarly on the far medial and lateral aspects, to replicate the native attachment of the plantar plate and collaterals. Two dedicated nonintersecting drill guides exist in the Hat-Trick (Smith and Nephew) system.

10. *Passing proximal phalanx sutures*: The plantar plate and collateral ligament sutures are passed from plantar to dorsal through the drill holes using a nitinol looped suture passer. If there is a longitudinal component to the plantar plate tear, it should be addressed.[9,35] Switching 1 limb of each plantar plate suture to the opposite hole crosses 2 sutures over the longitudinal tear.

11. *Tensioning the repair*: (If a Weil osteotomy was performed, this should be fixed to the desired length first. The pin-based distractor, if used, should also be

removed.) The MTP joint is held reduced in 20° of plantar flexion and the sutures are preliminarily tensioned over the dorsal bone bridge. The repair should be stressed with a drawer test. If satisfactory, final fixation can be completed by tying the sutures and/or with PEEK interference wires in the Hat-Trick (Smith and Nephew) system. The advantage of interference wires is that if the joint is not sufficiently stable after repair, the wires can be backed out and the sutures can be retensioned before wire reinsertion and final knot tying.

12. *Additional procedures:* A proximal interphalangeal resection arthroplasty or arthrodesis may be performed as indicated for distal deformity. The extensor tendons, if released, are Z-lengthened or transferred. A K-wire is not typically placed across the MTP joint, but with the postoperative dressing, the toe is placed in slight plantarflexion.

13. *Postoperative course:* Similar to other authors' instructions, patients are told to be weight bearing only through their heel in a stiff postoperative shoe for 6 weeks.[9,11,35] Active and passive range of motion exercises are begun at 6 weeks and, when comfortable, patients may advance to normal shoe wear. Other authors have reported results with earlier weight bearing and range of motion exercises.[10,12]

SUMMARY

Plantar plate tears are an underlying primary pathology that has previously been ignored in a number of lesser MTP diagnoses. Many previous solutions accommodated the loss of the plantar plate, and those techniques more than likely still have a large role. Attempting to restore the anatomic attachment of the plantar plate and collaterals, however, addresses the primary pathology. The evidence to date suggests that with appropriate indications, plantar plate repair is associated with improved pain scores and relatively high patient satisfaction.[10–12] Although indications and specific technique may vary from surgeon to surgeon, the dorsal approach to plantar plate repair should be included in the armamentarium when addressing lesser toe pathology.

REFERENCES

1. Thompson FM, Hamilton WG. Problems of the second metatarsophalangeal joint. Orthopedics 1987;10(1):83–9.
2. Doty JF, Coughlin MJ. Metatarsophalangeal joint instability of the lesser toes and plantar plate deficiency. J Am Acad Orthop Surg 2014;22(4):235–45.
3. Coughlin MJ, Schutt SA, Hirose CB, et al. Metatarsophalangeal joint pathology in crossover second toe deformity: a cadaveric study. Foot Ankle Int 2012;33(2): 133–40.
4. Deland JT, Lee KT, Sobel M, et al. Anatomy of the plantar plate and its attachments in the lesser metatarsal phalangeal joint. Foot Ankle Int 1995;16(8):480–6.
5. Johnston RB, Smith J, Daniels T. The plantar plate of the lesser toes: an anatomical study in human cadavers. Foot Ankle Int 1994;15(5):276–82.
6. Bhatia D, Myerson MS, Curtis MJ, et al. Anatomical restraints to dislocation of the second metatarsophalangeal joint and assessment of a repair technique. J Bone Joint Surg Am 1994;76(9):1371–5.
7. Chalayon O, Chertman C, Guss AD, et al. Role of plantar plate and surgical reconstruction techniques on static stability of lesser metatarsophalangeal joints: a biomechanical study. Foot Ankle Int 2013;34(10):1436–42.

8. Barg A, Courville XF, Nickisch F, et al. Role of collateral ligaments in metatarsophalangeal stability: a cadaver study. Foot Ankle Int 2012;33(10):877–82.

9. Nery C, Coughlin MJ, Baumfeld D, et al. Prospective evaluation of protocol for surgical treatment of lesser MTP joint plantar plate tears. Foot Ankle Int 2014; 35(9):876–85.

10. Weil L, Sung W, Weil LS, et al. Anatomic plantar plate repair using the Weil metatarsal osteotomy approach. Foot Ankle Spec 2011;4(3):145–50.

11. Flint WW, Macias DM, Jastifer JR, et al. Plantar plate repair for lesser metatarsophalangeal joint instability. Foot Ankle Int 2017;38(3):234–42.

12. Gregg J, Silberstein M, Clark C, et al. Plantar plate repair and Weil osteotomy for metatarsophalangeal joint instability. Foot Ankle Surg 2007;13(3):116–21.

13. Gregg JM, Silberstein M, Schneider T, et al. Sonography of plantar plates in cadavers: correlation with MRI and histology. AJR Am J Roentgenol 2006;186(4): 948–55.

14. Wang B, Guss A, Chalayon O, et al. Deep transverse metatarsal ligament and static stability of lesser metatarsophalangeal joints: a cadaveric study. Foot Ankle Int 2015;36(5):573–8.

15. Deland JT, Sobel M, Arnoczky SP, et al. Collateral ligament reconstruction of the unstable metatarsophalangeal joint: an in vitro study. Foot Ankle 1992;13(7): 391–5.

16. Klein EE, Weil L, Weil LS, et al. Clinical examination of plantar plate abnormality: a diagnostic perspective. Foot Ankle Int 2013;34(6):800–4.

17. Nery C, Coughlin MJ, Baumfeld D, et al. Lesser metatarsophalangeal joint instability: prospective evaluation and repair of plantar plate and capsular insufficiency. Foot Ankle Int 2012;33(4):301–11.

18. Nery C, Coughlin MJ, Baumfeld D, et al. MRI evaluation of the MTP plantar plates compared with arthroscopic findings: a prospective study. Foot Ankle Int 2013; 34(3):315–22.

19. Doty JF, Coughlin MJ, Weil L, et al. Etiology and management of lesser toe metatarsophalangeal joint instability. Foot Ankle Clin 2014;19(3):385–405.

20. Sung W, Weil L, Weil LS, et al. Diagnosis of plantar plate injury by magnetic resonance imaging with reference to intraoperative findings. J Foot Ankle Surg 2012; 51(5):570–4.

21. Yao L, Cracchiolo A, Farahani K, et al. Magnetic resonance imaging of plantar plate rupture. Foot Ankle Int 1996;17(1):33–6.

22. Yao L, Do HM, Cracchiolo A, et al. Plantar plate of the foot: findings on conventional arthrography and MR imaging. AJR Am J Roentgenol 1994;163(3):641–4.

23. Klein EE, Weil L, Weil LS, et al. Magnetic resonance imaging versus musculoskeletal ultrasound for identification and localization of plantar plate tears. Foot Ankle Spec 2012;5(6):359–65.

24. Gregg J, Silberstein M, Schneider T, et al. Sonographic and MRI evaluation of the plantar plate: a prospective study. Eur Radiol 2006;16(12):2661–9.

25. Powless SH, Elze ME. Metatarsophalangeal joint capsule tears: an analysis by arthrography, a new classification system and surgical management. J Foot Ankle Surg 2001;40(6):374–89.

26. Blitz NM, Ford LA, Christensen JC. Second metatarsophalangeal joint arthrography: a cadaveric correlation study. J Foot Ankle Surg 2004;43(4):231–40.

27. Mazzuca JW, Yonke B, Downes JM, et al. Fluoroscopic arthrography versus MR arthrography of the lesser metatarsophalangeal joints for the detection of tears of the plantar plate and joint capsule: a prospective comparative study. Foot Ankle Int 2013;34(2):200–9.

28. Trepman E, Yeo SJ. Nonoperative treatment of metatarsophalangeal joint synovitis. Foot Ankle Int 1995;16(12):771–7.
29. Mizel MS, Michelson JD. Nonsurgical treatment of monarticular nontraumatic synovitis of the second metatarsophalangeal joint. Foot Ankle Int 1997;18(7):424–6.
30. Peck CN, Macleod A, Barrie J. Lesser metatarsophalangeal instability: presentation, management, and outcomes. Foot Ankle Int 2012;33(7):565–70.
31. Bouché RT, Heit EJ. Combined plantar plate and hammertoe repair with flexor digitorum longus tendon transfer for chronic, severe sagittal plane instability of the lesser metatarsophalangeal joints: preliminary observations. J Foot Ankle Surg 2008;47(2):125–37.
32. Prissel MA, Hyer CF, Donovan JK, et al. Plantar plate repair using a direct plantar approach: an outcomes analysis. J Foot Ankle Surg 2017;56(3):434–9.
33. Cooper MT, Coughlin MJ. Sequential dissection for exposure of the second metatarsophalangeal joint. Foot Ankle Int 2011;32(3):294–9.
34. Jastifer JR, Coughlin MJ. Exposure via sequential release of the metatarsophalangeal joint for plantar plate repair through a dorsal approach without an intra-articular osteotomy. Foot Ankle Int 2015;36(3):335–8.
35. Watson TS, Reid DY, Frerichs TL. Dorsal approach for plantar plate repair with Weil osteotomy: operative technique. Foot Ankle Int 2014;35(7):730–9.
36. Clement RC, Eskildsen SM, Tennant JN. Technical tip and cost analysis for lesser toe plantar plate repair with a curved suture needle. Foot Ankle Int 2015;36(3):330–4.

Managing Complications of Lesser Toe and Metatarsophalangeal Joint Surgery

Phinit Phisitkul, MD

KEYWORDS

- Hammer toe • Claw toe • Complication • Lesser toe • Revision
- Metatarsophalangeal • MTP

KEY POINTS

- Lesser toe surgeries are challenging and require meticulous techniques.
- When complications occur, understanding of the culprits and proper execution of treatments are essential.
- There is high propensity for the metatarsophalangeal joint to develop hyperextension deformity.
- Patients should be provided with realistic expectations for lesser toe reconstructive procedures.

INTRODUCTION

Surgeries for the lesser toe and metatarsophalangeal (MTP) joint are among the top procedures performed in the foot and ankle according to the Medicare database, leading to an estimation of total economic burden of more than $1 billion in 2011.[1] However, there is a paucity of high-quality outcome studies in the literature to guide medical practice. Patients usually seek care for their feet from various types of providers, including physical therapists, orthotists, podiatrists, family physicians, and orthopedic surgeons, leading to nonuniform treatment strategies. With the growing number of surgeries performed to correct lesser toe deformities, surgeons should be familiar with the potential complications and the strategies to manage each of them appropriately. This article combines the authors' experience with the best available evidence in the literature to cover a spectrum of potential complications of surgeries on the lesser toe and MTP joint.

Challenges are recognized for the treatment of lesser toe conditions because of the lack of standardized terminology, anatomic susceptibility for developing hyperextension deformity at the MTP joint, close relationship with the hallux and more

The author has nothing to disclose.
Private practice, 942 Forest Edge Cir, Coralville 52241, USA
E-mail address: Phinit-phisitkul@uiowa.edu

proximal malalignments, long-standing deformity, and the requirement of delicate bone and soft tissue handling. There is no universal distinction between the term hammer toe and claw toe, making it difficult to categorize outcomes and complications with accurate diagnoses.[2] For the simplification purposes, the author defines the deformity at each joint as rigid or flexible to avoid the overuse of the conflicting terms.

Potential complications of the lesser toe surgeries are divided into the following 4 categories:

1. Wound and soft tissue
2. Malalignment
3. Neurologic
4. Fixation and hardware

WOUND AND SOFT TISSUE
Toe Gangrene

This rare but serious complication can occur after an extensive toe deformity correction, especially in elderly patients with long-standing conditions or smokers.[3] Often patients may have underlying vascular impairment or Reynaud phenomenon. It is important that a risk of toe amputation is discussed with the patient during the informed consent process when significant realignment of the MTP or proximal interphalangeal (PIP) joint is required. A risk of toe amputation was found to be 0.4% from a large series by Kramer and colleagues[4] on 2698 hammer toes. Surgeons should make it a routine to check for the return of capillary refill after the deflation of tourniquet. A toe with sluggish return of normal "pinkish" color may be warmed up using gauze soaked with warm saline. Lack of improvement after 25 to 30 minutes of observation should alert further interventions including removal of Kirschner (K)-wire, loosening of flexor tendon transfer, application of loose dressing, and discussion with the patient and/or family. The toe that developed dry gangrene should be allowed to demarcate before a definitive amputation at a later date (**Fig. 1**).[5]

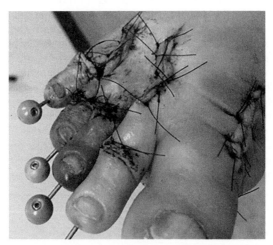

Fig. 1. Clinical picture of dry gangrene developed in a patient with multiple comorbidities after a rheumatoid forefoot reconstruction. Further observation allowed demarcation of necrotic tissue and partial toe amputations were performed.

Wound Infection

Wound infection is one of the most common postsurgical complications in the forefoot due to bacterial colonization, sweating, inadequate blood supply, degree of soft tissue dissection, and lack of postoperative compliance. Patients might have underlying diabetes with poor control or a history of nicotine use. As most of the forefoot procedures are performed as outpatient procedures, patients and/or family need to be educated about observation for symptoms and signs of infection, including increasing pain or throbbing, increasing wound drainage, and fever or chills. Kramer and colleagues[4] found the frequency of prescribing antibiotics at follow-up to be 11%, whereas a significant pin-tract infection occurred in only 0.3%. Surgeons should have low threshold in the indication for wound irrigation and debridement when abscess formation is suspected. However, most of concerns about wound infection could be resolved by strict elevation and oral antibiotics. Partial necrosis of overlying soft tissue usually can be observed until deep tissue healing has occurred and the necrotic tissue sloughs off with wet to dry dressing or a surgical debridement. Wound dehiscence associated with infection should not be surgically closed but allowed to granulate from inside out from wound packing. When chemical debridement is required, silver sulfadiazine or 0.25% acetic acid can be added to the packing gauge to inhibit bacterial growth.[6] In cases with fulminant osteomyelitis, an adequate surgical debridement is required to eradicate infection ranging from partial bone resection to a toe or a ray amputation. Bone voids in the zone of infection can be filled with antibiotic impregnated cement or calcium sulfate pellets.[7]

Stiffness

Stiffness on its own should not be considered a complication for lesser toe surgeries. Most of the surgeries on the lesser toe and the MTP joint will create more or less stiffness and patients should be well informed about this condition before surgery. Certain types of procedure, such as PIP fusion, distal interphalangeal joint (DIP) fusion, MTP stabilization, or flexor to extensor transfer tendon transfer (FETT) will essentially create more stiffness in the operated toe to relieve pain and correct deformity.[8] Although rare, degenerative change can also develop after surgical reconstructions at the MTP joint. If the MTP joint is arthritic or avascular/necrotic, a resection arthroplasty with or without tendon allograft interposition may be considered (**Fig. 2**). There is insufficient evidence for the use of resurfacing implant in the revision settings. The most problematic stiffness is when the MTP joint is contracted into hyperextension posture without

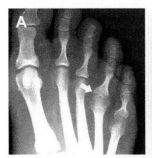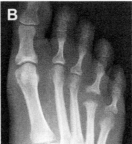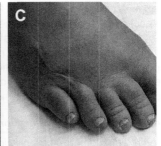

Fig. 2. Preoperative radiograph (A) demonstrated a patient with floating right fourth toe with arthritis (arrow). Resection arthroplasty with tendon allograft interposition was performed. Postoperative radiograph (B) and clinical picture (C) at 3 months are demonstrated.

adequate plantarflexion. The patients should be educated to perform active and passive plantarflexion exercise of the MTP joint when possible for any surgery in the lesser toes to prevent this occurrence. The management of this condition is described in detail in the next section.

MALALIGNMENT
Floating Toe

Floating toe is considered the most common complication or residual deformity after a Weil osteotomy, and has been reported at an average of 36%.[9] It has been found to be more common in cases with an associated PIP fusion.[10] This condition could be explained at least partly by the change in the axis of rotation of the MTP joint and partly by the loss of tension of the plantar plate and plantar fascia insertions due to shortening.[11] Most of the floating toes are fortunately asymptomatic and a revision surgery is not required. Patients with mild symptoms may be treated with custom insoles with a relief at the metatarsal head or with toe taping into more plantarflexion. If nonoperative measures fail, a surgical treatment may be considered. The first consideration is whether there is any osseous deformity and if the MTP joint is viable. Plantar prominence secondary to the configuration of the Weil osteotomy may be treated with a dorsal closing wedge osteotomy at the proximal metatarsal. In any case, there should be an attempt to create plantarflexion force at the proximal phalange. This can be achieved by a plantar plate repair and/or FETT or a modified flexor digitorum longus transfer.[12] Lee and colleagues[13] demonstrated the possibility of using the flexor digitorum brevis transfer to prevent floating toe deformity after a Weil osteotomy.

Extension Contracture

Contracture of the MTP joint is perhaps the most common disabling condition following a lesser toe surgery. It could occur from the bony malalignment, inadequate soft tissue balancing, or postoperative immobilization. First line of management includes physical therapy for stretching exercise of the dorsal soft tissue, an insole with a relief underneath the affected metatarsal head, and Achilles tendon stretching exercise. Plantarflexion deformity of the involved ray from a cavovarus deformity or from plantar displacement of Weil osteotomy accentuates the hyperextension posture of the joint. The presence of plantarflexion deformity of the metatarsal may be corrected by a dorsal closing wedge osteotomy at the proximal metatarsal.[14] When addressing dorsal soft tissue contracture, a complete release or preferably excision of both extensor tendons together with dorsal joint capsule is crucial.[15] If the toe continues to be elevated on a simulated weight-bearing position, an FETT is recommended as an additional step (**Fig. 3**). As the FETT is held only with sutures on the dorsal aspect of the proximal phalange, K-wire fixation across the MTP joint in slight plantarflexion may provide additional stability for 6 weeks until the tendon transfer is healed. It is important that the deformity must be completely corrected with soft tissue or bony procedures before K-wire fixation. An incomplete correction of deformity will quickly recur after K-wire removal. If dorsal skin contracture was found to be a deforming force, addition of Z-plasty to the skin incision may be helpful.[16]

Joint Subluxation or Dislocation

Dorsal subluxation or dislocation of the MTP joint can occur when a toe deformity correction is performed without anatomic repair of the plantar plate and collateral ligaments or when the repair is deficient due to a long-standing deformity or multiple cortisone injections.[17] This condition may or may not cause symptoms depending

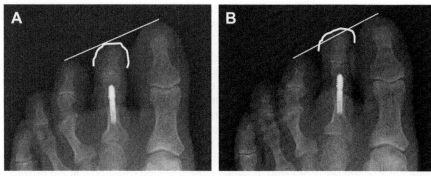

Fig. 3. Preoperative (*A*) and postoperative (*B*) anteroposterior radiographs of a patient who developed extension contracture of the second MTP joint after a PIP fusion with complete loss of toe purchase. A complete extensor tendon and dorsal capsule transection together with flexor tendon transfer was performed in the revision procedure. A relatively longer second toe is appreciated due to the flattening of the toe after correction of extension contracture.

on the presence of overloading problems at the metatarsal head. Patients with hallux valgus deformity and unstable first ray are susceptible to overloading of the second MTP joint. This is even more profound when the second metatarsal is relatively longer than adjacent rays. Initial management includes the use of custom insoles with a relief underneath the affected metatarsal head. Medial forefoot posting may be appropriate if an unstable first ray coexists. Patients may also benefit from Achilles tendon stretching exercise. When nonsurgical treatments fail, surgical treatment can be considered. Conditions leading to overloading of the lesser metatarsal head should be addressed, such as gastrocnemius recession for equinus contracture, hallux valgus correction to stabilize the first ray, and Weil osteotomy for long lesser metatarsals (**Fig. 4**). In patients without prior plantar plate repair or FETT, these reconstructive options may be indicated.[17] In patients with prior plantar plate repair or FETT, resection arthroplasty of the affected metatarsal head with or without tendon allograft may help alleviate pain from plantar overloading but the toe alignment is unpredictable.[18]

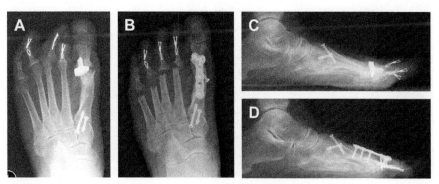

Fig. 4. Preoperative (*A, C*) and postoperative (*B, D*) radiographs of a 50-year-old patient with rheumatoid arthritis who has severe metatarsalgia after 2 surgical procedures. Gastrocnemius recession, arthrodesis of the first MTP joint, and resection arthroplasty of the lesser metatarsal heads were performed in the revision procedure.

Alternatively, an amputation of the affected toe with or without partial metatarsal head resection may be considered as the last resort.[19]

Transfer Metatarsalgia

This condition occurs due to an uneven weight-bearing surface in the forefoot after a bony realignment, such as Weil osteotomy, metatarsal head resection, or elevation of a ray from an osteotomy or fusion.[9] Patients with other mechanically overloading causes, such as obesity, equinus contracture, planovalgus deformity, or unstable first ray, are more susceptible to this complication. Patients with mild symptoms could be treated with orthoses such as custom insole to offload the prominence. Isolated prominent metatarsal head can be corrected with a plantar condylectomy.[20] If more elevation of the affected ray is required, a dorsal closing wedge osteotomy at the proximal metatarsal is indicated.[14] When the imbalance in weight transfer is related to deficiency of the first ray, early correction with realignment osteotomy or fusion to allow more weight-bearing at the first ray can help relieve pain and potentially prevent permanent damage to the second and third metatarsophalangeal joints. If the cascade of lesser metatarsals is disrupted, as shown in anterior posterior radiographs, a Weil osteotomy of the long metatarsals is appropriate (**Fig. 5**).[21] Occasionally, shortening of all the lesser metatarsals is required to create balance in the forefoot. In patients with evidence of forefoot overloading together with gastrocnemius or gastrocsoleus contracture, a lengthening procedure can be considered.[22]

Coronal Plane Deformity

Coronal plane deformity can occur from multiple factors related to imbalance at the lesser MTP joint. The hallmark of this deformity is the association of plantar plate

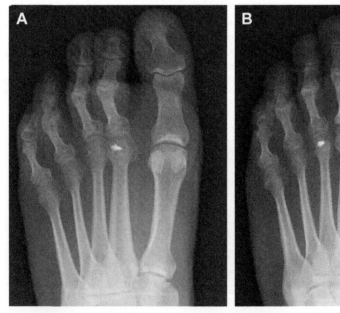

Fig. 5. Preoperative (A) and postoperative (B) anteroposterior radiographs of a patient who developed transfer metatarsalgia at the third metatarsal head and residual extension contracture of the second MTP joint. Weil osteotomy of the third metatarsal head and second MTP plantar plate repair were performed in the revision procedure.

and collateral ligaments injury.[23] The understanding of coronal plane balance is evolving and the patients will need to be counseled that perfectly looking toes may not always be achievable. The connection between the bases of the adjacent proximal phalanges through the deep transverse intermetatarsal ligament, natatory ligament, and Moore ligament can cause second and third MTP joints to drift medially as the hallux valgus is progressing or recurring. Mediolateral translation of the lesser metatarsal head can cause a deviation of the proximal phalange in the opposite direction.[24] Contracture of the extrinsic tendons can aggravate the deviation as the deforming force if the deformity is more evident. The most important culprit of coronal plane deformity is a failure to repair the plantar plate and collateral ligament or a failure of the repair construct. Patients with mild symptoms may be treated with silicone toe spacers, toe crests, or taping. In a low-demand patient or when extensive surgeries have failed, a toe amputation at the level of the MTP joint will provide generally very good results and early weight-bearing (**Fig. 6**). Additional decompression of the plantar condyle may be required if the affected metatarsal head remains prominent on examination after the toe amputation. When a revision surgery is contemplated, the surgeon should consider correcting both the primary pathology, for example, plantar plate and collateral ligament tear and contributing factors such as hallux valgus deformity, lesser metatarsal deformity, and extrinsic tendon contracture.[25,26]

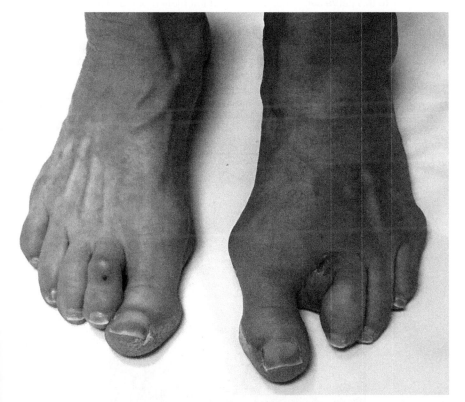

Fig. 6. Clinical picture of a patient 6 weeks after a left second toe amputation is shown. The patient has been doing heel weight-bearing for 2 weeks followed by walking as tolerated in normal shoes.

Plantar plate can be approached from plantar, dorsal, or intermetatarsal incisions.[27–29] Plantar incisions have some reservations because of potentially painful scar and inability to address other structures, such as capsular contracture, collateral ligaments, and metatarsal bones. Dorsal incisions can address a single MTP joint very well but the approach does require a complete release of both collateral ligaments and the plantar plate. The intermetatarsal approach allows exposure to 2 adjacent MTP joints and can address the plantar plate and ipsilateral collateral ligament without a complete joint stripping (**Fig. 7**). The repair of plantar plate and collateral ligaments can be achieved using free-hand techniques or commercially available repair kits. When the plantar plate repair is insufficient due to long-standing deformity with attenuated soft tissue and possible prior cortisone injections, augmentation with a flexor tendon transfer is recommended.[18] Deficiency of the collateral ligament can be reinforced using an extensor digitorum brevis transfer.[30]

NEUROLOGIC
Postsurgical Neuroma

Damage to the sensory nerve branches to the toe can be catastrophic to the surgical outcome. The dorsal cutaneous nerve branches are quite small and a meticulous surgical approach with gentle soft tissue retraction is required. On the plantar aspect, the intermetatarsal nerve is located just plantar to the deep transverse intermetatarsal ligament. Injury to this nerve can occur during a plantar plate repair or extensor digitorum brevis transfer underneath the deep transverse intermetatarsal ligament. Most of the symptoms from postsurgical neuritis resolve over time. Physical therapy, insoles, and gabapentin can be used to alleviate pain. Cortisone injections can be used for symptomatic treatment but multiple injections can lead to soft tissue atrophy. In recalcitrant cases, a diagnostic injection under ultrasound guidance may help confirm the diagnosis.[31] Injured intermetatarsal nerves can be explored using a previous dorsal incision. The neuroma should be identified and excised. The proximal nerve stump is then transferred into intrinsic muscles in the arch of foot.[32]

Complex Regional Pain Syndrome Type 1

The occurrence of complex regional pain syndrome (CRPS) type 1 can lead to severe disabling pain that requires intensive therapy. It has been found to occur in 4% of

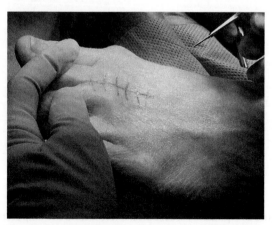

Fig. 7. Skin incision for the intermetatarsal approach is marked for the correction of plantar plate injury of the second and third MTP joints.

patients undergoing elective foot and ankle surgery.[33] This condition should be distinguished from the postsurgical neuroma, as further surgical treatment is not indicated. Pain from CRPS type 1 is not limited to the neural anatomy of damage nerves. Failure to relieve pain from an ultrasound-guided diagnostic injection to the suspected nerve injury suggests the presence of this condition. Patients should be treated using a multimodal approach, including physical therapy, psychiatric evaluation, gabapentin, nutritional supplementation, and possibly a referral to a pain specialist.[34]

FIXATION OR HARDWARE
Nonunion

Nonunion can occur from multiple treatment modalities for the lesser toe deformities including DIP fusion, PIP fusion, proximal phalangeal osteotomy, and various locations for metatarsal osteotomy.[35] Generally, fibrous healing at the PIP joint level yields satisfactory outcomes.[36] Nonunion at the DIP joint fusion without a flexion contracture is also well tolerated.[37] Nonunion of the metatarsal osteotomy is uncommon but can become symptomatic necessitating a revision surgery.[38] As a general rule, the patient undergoing a fusion surgery should be evaluated for a potential vitamin D deficiency and appropriately treated with high-dose supplementation. Patients should refrain from nicotine products at least a month before surgery. Each fusion surface should be debrided thoroughly followed by drilling of the subchondral bone. Fluid irrigation is essential during an osteotomy to minimize thermal necrosis of the bone. When a

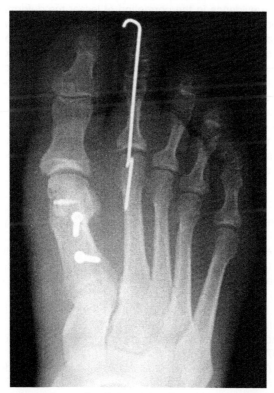

Fig. 8. Anteroposterior radiograph of the right foot demonstrates a breakage of the 0.045-inch K-wire at the level of the second MTP joint.

nonunion is symptomatic, an orthosis to offload and immobilize the digit should be considered. Osteosynthesis of the nonunion around the lesser rays can be achieved using rigid fixation with implants and augmentation with autologous bone graft.

Kirschner-Wire Breakage

K-wire breakage is a potential complication that may lead to failure of surgery. When the break occurs early in the recovery phase and especially if a part of the K-wire is left within the MTP joint, a revision surgery to remove the broken wire pieces and to replace them with another K-wire may be indicated. It is important that surgeons use at least 0.062-inch K-wires for pinning in the toe and the MTP joint to minimize this risk (**Fig. 8**).[39] K-wires must not be used to lever against an uncorrected deforming force, as the deformity will predictably recur after the wire removal or an early wire breakage may occur. Although earlier K-wire removal may help avoiding breakage, sufficient soft tissue and bone stabilization usually occurs after 4 to 6 weeks.[40] If the patient is asymptomatic, the broken part of the K-wire that is not irritating the MTP joint can be left alone. K-wire removal from the medullary canal of a metatarsal bone can be achieved by making a small cortical window proximally to push the K-wire out through the MTP joint.

SUMMARY

The anatomy of the lesser toes is highly complicated and not yet well understood. The high propensity of the MTP joint to develop hyperextension deformity should be recognized. As the evidence in the correction of lesser toe deformity is developed, a treatment should be designed with the concern of potential complications. Surgeons should provide each patient with a realistic expectation for lesser toe reconstructive procedures. A successful surgical result requires a well-planned procedure, accurate execution using proper techniques, and meticulous postoperative care. The patient and the care team should be clearly informed once a complication has occurred. Most of the complications in lesser toe surgeries do not require a revision surgery but lengthy and labor-intensive clinical visits are the rule. When there is a doubt in the predictability of a revision procedure, a second opinion or a referral should be done early rather than after multiple failed attempts. It is always advisable for medical doctors to exercise the most important principle for a surgical practice, "Primum non nocere" or "first, do no harm."

REFERENCES

1. Belatti DA, Phisitkul P. Economic burden of foot and ankle surgery in the US Medicare population. Foot Ankle Int 2014;35(4):334–40.
2. Schrier JC, Verheyen CC, Louwerens JW. Definitions of hammer toe and claw toe: an evaluation of the literature. J Am Podiatr Med Assoc 2009;99(3):194–7.
3. Solan MC, Davies MS. Revision surgery of the lesser toes. Foot Ankle Clin 2011; 16(4):621–45.
4. Kramer WC, Parman M, Marks RM. Hammertoe correction with k-wire fixation. Foot Ankle Int 2015;36(5):494–502.
5. Walden R, Adar R, Mozes M. Gangrene of toes with normal peripheral pulses. Ann Surg 1977;185(3):269–72.
6. Williams RL, Ayre WN, Khan WS, et al. Acetic acid as part of a debridement protocol during revision total knee arthroplasty. J Arthroplasty 2017;32(3):953–7.
7. McNally MA, Ferguson JY, Lau AC, et al. Single-stage treatment of chronic osteomyelitis with a new absorbable, gentamicin-loaded, calcium sulphate/hydroxyapatite

biocomposite: a prospective series of 100 cases. Bone Joint J 2016;98-B(9): 1289–96.

8. Myerson MS, Jung HG. The role of toe flexor-to-extensor transfer in correcting metatarsophalangeal joint instability of the second toe. Foot Ankle Int 2005; 26(9):675–9.

9. Highlander P, VonHerbulis E, Gonzalez A, et al. Complications of the Weil osteotomy. Foot Ankle Spec 2011;4(3):165–70.

10. Migues A, Slullitel G, Bilbao F, et al. Floating-toe deformity as a complication of the Weil osteotomy. Foot Ankle Int 2004;25(9):609–13.

11. Perez HR, Reber LK, Christensen JC. The role of passive plantar flexion in floating toes following Weil osteotomy. J Foot Ankle Surg 2008;47(6):520–6.

12. Rippstein PF, Park YU. A modified technique for flexor-to-extensor tendon transfer to correct residual metatarsophalangeal extension in the treatment of hammertoes. J Foot Ankle Surg 2014;53(6):810–2.

13. Lee LC, Charlton TP, Thordarson DB. Flexor digitorum brevis transfer for floating toe prevention after Weil osteotomy: a cadaveric study. Foot Ankle Int 2013; 34(12):1724–8.

14. Barouk LS. The BRT proximal metatarsal osteotomy. In: Barouk LS, editor. Forefoot reconstruction. Paris: Springer Paris; 2005. p. 139–54.

15. Frey S, Helix-Giordanino M, Piclet-Legre B. Percutaneous correction of second toe proximal deformity: proximal interphalangeal release, flexor digitorum brevis tenotomy and proximal phalanx osteotomy. Orthop Traumatol Surg Res 2015; 101(6):753–8.

16. Myerson MS, Fortin P, Girard P. Use of skin Z-plasty for management of extension contracture in recurrent claw- and hammertoe deformity. Foot Ankle Int 1994; 15(4):209–12.

17. Shima H, Okuda R, Yasuda T, et al. Surgical reduction and ligament reconstruction for chronic dorsal dislocation of the lesser metatarsophalangeal joint associated with hallux valgus. J Orthop Sci 2015;20(6):1019–29.

18. Bouche RT, Heit EJ. Combined plantar plate and hammertoe repair with flexor digitorum longus tendon transfer for chronic, severe sagittal plane instability of the lesser metatarsophalangeal joints: preliminary observations. J Foot Ankle Surg 2008;47(2):125–37.

19. Gallentine JW, DeOrio JK. Removal of the second toe for severe hammertoe deformity in elderly patients. Foot Ankle Int 2005;26(5):353–8.

20. Marx R, Mizel MS. Technique tip: a modified technique for plantar DuVries condylectomy. Foot Ankle Int 2007;28(12):1301.

21. Barouk LS. Weil's metatarsal osteotomy in the treatment of metatarsalgia. Orthopade 1996;25(4):338–44 [in German].

22. Abdulmassih S, Phisitkul P, Femino JE, et al. Triceps surae contracture: implications for foot and ankle surgery. J Am Acad Orthop Surg 2013;21(7):398–407.

23. Deland JT, Sung IH. The medial crosssover toe: a cadaveric dissection. Foot Ankle Int 2000;21(5):375–8.

24. Klinge SA, McClure P, Fellars T, et al. Modification of the Weil/Maceira metatarsal osteotomy for coronal plane malalignment during crossover toe correction: case series. Foot Ankle Int 2014;35(6):584–91.

25. Gougoulias N, Sakellariou A. Proximal closing wedge lesser metatarsal osteotomy for metatarsophalangeal joint transverse plane realignment. Surgical technique and outcome. Foot Ankle Surg 2014;20(1):30–3.

26. Flint WW, Macias DM, Jastifer JR, et al. Plantar plate repair for lesser metatarsophalangeal joint instability. Foot Ankle Int 2017;38(3):234–42.

27. McAlister JE, Hyer CF. The direct plantar plate repair technique. Foot Ankle Spec 2013;6(6):446–51.

28. Phisitkul P, Hosuru Siddappa V, Sittapairoj T, et al. Cadaveric evaluation of dorsal intermetatarsal approach for plantar plate and lateral collateral ligament repair of the lesser metatarsophalangeal joints. Foot Ankle Int 2017;38(7):791–6.

29. Nery C, Coughlin MJ, Baumfeld D, et al. Prospective evaluation of protocol for surgical treatment of lesser MTP joint plantar plate tears. Foot Ankle Int 2014; 35(9):876–85.

30. Ellis SJ, Young E, Endo Y, et al. Correction of multiplanar deformity of the second toe with metatarsophalangeal release and extensor brevis reconstruction. Foot Ankle Int 2013;34(6):792–9.

31. Ata AM, Onat SS, Ozcakar L. Ultrasound-guided diagnosis and treatment of Morton's neuroma. Pain Physician 2016;19(2):E355–8.

32. Rungprai C, Cychosz CC, Phruetthiphat O, et al. Simple neurectomy versus neurectomy with intramuscular implantation for interdigital neuroma: a comparative study. Foot Ankle Int 2015;36(12):1412–24.

33. Rewhorn MJ, Leung AH, Gillespie A, et al. Incidence of complex regional pain syndrome after foot and ankle surgery. J Foot Ankle Surg 2014;53(3):256–8.

34. Lee KJ, Kirchner JS. Complex regional pain syndrome and chronic pain management in the lower extremity. Foot Ankle Clin 2002;7(2):409–19.

35. Haque S, Kakwani R, Chadwick C, et al. Outcome of minimally invasive distal metatarsal metaphyseal osteotomy (DMMO) for lesser toe metatarsalgia. Foot Ankle Int 2016;37(1):58–63.

36. Catena F, Doty JF, Jastifer J, et al. Prospective study of hammertoe correction with an intramedullary implant. Foot Ankle Int 2014;35(4):319–25.

37. Coughlin MJ. Operative repair of the mallet toe deformity. Foot Ankle Int 1995; 16(3):109–16.

38. Herzog JL, Goforth WD, Stone PA, et al. A modified fixation technique for a decompressional shortening osteotomy: a retrospective analysis. J Foot Ankle Surg 2014;53(2):131–6.

39. Zingas C, Katcherian DA, Wu KK. Kirschner wire breakage after surgery of the lesser toes. Foot Ankle Int 1995;16(8):504–9.

40. Klammer G, Baumann G, Moor BK, et al. Early complications and recurrence rates after Kirschner wire transfixion in lesser toe surgery: a prospective randomized study. Foot Ankle Int 2012;33(2):105–12.

Treatment of Freiberg Disease

Jeffrey D. Seybold, MD[a],*, Jacob R. Zide, MD[b]

KEYWORDS

- Freiberg disease • Avascular necrosis • Metatarsal • Osteotomy
- Interpositional arthroplasty

KEY POINTS

- Freiberg disease, or osteochondrosis of the lesser metatarsal head, most commonly involves the second metatarsal and typically presents during the second or third decades of life.
- The most commonly used staging system effectively identifies cases in which normal joint anatomy can be restored.
- Conservative measures that limit overload of the affected metatarsal head are the first-line treatments in all stages of Freiberg disease, with high success rates for Smillie stage I to III disease.
- Operative treatments are divided into joint-preserving and joint-reconstructing procedures. Although multiple case series describe success with numerous techniques, there are no currently established guidelines for treatment.
- In general, joint debridement with a metatarsal osteotomy is preferred for Smillie stage II to III disease; joint debridement with interpositional arthroplasty is reserved for stage IV and V disease.

INTRODUCTION

The first reported treatment of Freiberg disease was described by the eponymous Dr. Albert H. Freiberg[1] in 1914. In his account of 6 cases, he reported that 4 patients were managed conservatively, whereas 2 required metatarsophalangeal (MTP) joint arthrotomy with removal of loose bodies.

Conservative measures are the first line of treatment when managing symptomatic Freiberg disease. When nonsurgical strategies fail, a wide variety of surgical alternatives have been reported. However, guiding the patient toward the appropriate surgery

Disclosure: The authors have nothing to disclose.
[a] Twin Cities Orthopedics, 4010 West 65th Street, Edina, MN 55435, USA; [b] Department of Orthopaedic Surgery, Baylor University Medical Center, 3500 Gaston Avenue, Dallas, TX 75246, USA
* Corresponding author.
E-mail address: jseybold@tcomn.com

Foot Ankle Clin N Am 23 (2018) 157–169
https://doi.org/10.1016/j.fcl.2017.09.011

foot.theclinics.com

can be challenging because most of these options are based on small case series and no validated algorithm exists to help guide surgeons in their decision making. This article provides an update regarding available treatments and support for their use in the management of Freiberg disease.

CLINICAL AND RADIOGRAPHIC EVALUATION
Clinical Evaluation

The peak age at the onset of symptoms is within the second decade of life. Patients usually present with pain localized to the affected MTP joint. They may recall a traumatic event involving the foot or the pain may simply arise without an obvious injury to the forefoot. Barefoot walking and wearing shoes with an elevated heel often amplify the symptoms because increased pressure is placed on the metatarsal head. Symptoms typically involve a single metatarsal and bilateral involvement is present in less than 10% of cases.[2] The second metatarsal is most commonly affected, comprising approximately two-thirds of all cases, with the third metatarsal involved in 27%.[3]

Examination of the affected MTP joint generally reveals an effusion and surrounding swelling. This swelling is frequently seen as a loss of the normal contour of the extensor tendons to the toe. The MTP joint is tender to palpation and range of motion is often diminished. Pain generally diminishes quickly as palpation is performed away from the joint. There may be palpable grinding with passive joint motion depending on the severity of arthritic change present. As the disease process progresses, coronal and/or sagittal plane deformity may develop, with a clinical appearance similar to a claw toe or crossover toe.

Radiographic Evaluation

Standard radiographic evaluation begins with standard 3-view weight-bearing images of the foot (anteroposterior, oblique, and lateral). Early in the disease process, typically within 3 to 6 weeks of the onset of symptoms, the joint and osseous structures may look normal aside from subtle widening of the joint space.[4] As the disease progresses, flattening of the metatarsal head and increased subchondral bone density are noted.[2,5] Anteroposterior radiographs may appear unremarkable in early disease with flattening of the dorsal metatarsal head only noted on the oblique view. Over time, additional findings include loose bodies in the joint, progressive narrowing of the joint space, and metatarsal head sclerosis.[6]

In more subtle or inconclusive cases, MRI may be helpful in confirming the diagnosis. Osteonecrosis of the metatarsal head on the MRI classically appears hypointense on T1-weighted images with a mix of low and high signal intensity on T2-weighted images.[7]

STAGING

Several staging and classification systems are available to describe changes and offer treatment suggestions for Freiberg disease.[3,6,8] The classic 1966 staging system by Smillie[6] describes the structural changes of the metatarsal head observed intraoperatively, although many of the pathologic findings are evident radiographically. This system is the most commonly referenced in outcomes studies and is outlined in **Box 1**.

NONOPERATIVE MANAGEMENT

Nonoperative management should be first line of treatment regardless of the severity of disease at the time of presentation. Strategies for conservative treatment include

---

Box 1
Smillie staging system for Freiberg disease

- Stage I: a fissure fracture in the ischemic epiphysis. Cancellous bone at the fracture appears sclerotic. Compared with the adjacent metaphysis, the epiphysis shows absence of blood supply.

- Stage II: absorption of cancellous bone occurs proximally. The central cartilage sinks into the head while the margins and plantar cartilage remain intact. This process results in an altered contour of the articular surface.

- Stage III: further absorption occurs and the central portion sinks deeper, creating larger projections on either side. The plantar cartilage remains intact.

- Stage IV: the central portion continues to sink such that the plantar hinge gives way. The peripheral projections fracture and fold over the central portion. Restoration of the anatomy is no longer possible.

- Stage V: the final stage shows arthrosis with flattening and deformity of the metatarsal head. Only the plantar portion of the metatarsal cartilage retains the original contour of the head. Loose bodies have reduced in size and the shaft of the metatarsal is thickened and dense.

Data from Smillie IS. Treatment of Freiberg's infraction. Proc R Soc Med 1967;60(1):29–31.

---

use of oral antiinflammatory medications, avoidance of high-impact activity (such as running and jumping), and modification of shoewear. Use of a stiff-soled shoe with a rocker bottom can be helpful to offload the forefoot during toe-off. Alternatively, orthotics with a metatarsal pad or bar can be used to relieve pressure under the metatarsal heads. In acute presentations with more intense pain, a period of immobilization and/or non–weight bearing with a cast, boot, or hard-soled shoe for up to 6 weeks may be advantageous. Most patients with Smillie stage I to III disease respond well to conservative treatment measures with long-term success (**Fig. 1**).[9]

OPERATIVE MANAGEMENT

A myriad of case reports can be found regarding operative treatment of Freiberg disease. These procedures are typically entertained for advanced stages of disease at initial presentation (Smillie IV–V) or after failure of the conservative measures in the early stages of the disease (Smillie I–III). There is little consensus as to the best treatment option, although general recommendations can be made based on the stage of disease at the time of intervention. Grade B recommendations have been provided for the use of joint debridement and joint-sparing osteotomies for nearly all stages of Freiberg infraction, as well as for limited excision of periarticular tissue with interpositional arthroplasty for Smillie IV to V disease.[5]

Joint-Sparing Procedures

Joint-sparing procedures are typically reserved for Smillie stages I to III when there is at least some preserved plantar chondral surface and contour. Although not immune to complications such as transfer metatarsalgia and subsequent MTP joint stiffness and deformity, these risks are mitigated if care is taken not to dramatically alter the MTP joint anatomy.

Joint debridement
Debridement of the MTP joint is typically performed in conjunction with the other procedures described later. Adequate debridement of the joint includes removal of any

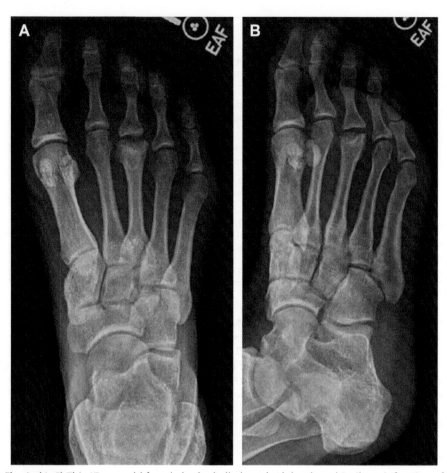

Fig. 1. (*A, B*) This 17-year-old female basketball player had developed Freiberg infraction of the second metatarsal at the age of 12 years. She presented with increasing pain localized to the third MTP joint. Smillie stage II disease was noted on radiographic imaging. The patient was managed conservatively with boot immobilization initially and has subsequently returned to play using a carbon fiber plate insert. Note the fairly normal appearance of the second metatarsal head.

loose bodies and prominent osteophytes, hypertrophic synovium, and delaminated areas of cartilage. Originally described by Freiberg,[1] joint debridement has been met with good success.[1,6,9–11] Smillie[6] supported the value of debridement in his original series. Sproul and colleagues[11] evaluated the effects of joint debridement in 10 patients with varying degrees of athletic activity. All patients noted improvement in symptoms with restoration of 80% normal range of motion. Arthroscopic debridement has also been described in 2 case reports[12,13]; both patients remained symptom free after the procedure.

Core decompression
The concepts of core decompression have been well used in the hip, but few reports have been described using this technique in Freiberg disease.[14,15] The goal of the technique is to relieve increased intraosseous pressure in the avascular bone at the

metatarsal head, allowing revascularization and healing of bone and the overlying chondral surface. Two case reports[14,15] have described the use of core decompression for patients with early-stage disease, before structural changes were noted at the metatarsal head. A 1.1-mm Kirschner wire was used to fenestrate the metatarsal head multiple times. Patients all noted complete relief of pain and did not show progressive structural changes. This technique may provide good results in combination with joint debridement for Smillie stage I disease (**Fig. 2**).

Grafting procedures
Grafting of bone at the diseased metatarsal head was first described by Smillie[6] in 1967. A 14-mm by 5-mm slot is created in the dorsum of the metatarsal head, at the border of the epiphysis and metaphysis. For stage I and II disease, the author simply perforated the epiphyseal plate in multiple locations to restore blood flow across the sclerotic bone. In stage III disease, the collapsed portion of the metatarsal head was reduced and the epiphyseal plate once again perforated. The defect left after reduction of the metatarsal head and the slot was backfilled with cancellous autograft bone.

A similar technique was described by Lawton[16] in 1979 in which autogenous bone graft is used to complete an epiphysiodesis, effectively eliminating the dead, sclerotic bone at the epiphysis and allowing restoration of blood flow to the subchondral bone. Helal and Gibb[9] used bone grafting in Smillie grade I and II disease, with complete symptom relief and restoration of normal radiographic appearance of the metatarsal head in 8 of 11 patients. Two patients noted postoperative pain solely with impact activity and wearing high-heeled shoes. The investigators also used a Kirschner wire to stabilize the metatarsal head postoperatively and protected the foot in a walking plaster cast for 6 weeks.

Transplant of an osteochondral plug from the femoral condyle was first described by Hayashi and colleagues[17] in a patient with Smillie stage IV disease. The patient returned to running and athletic activity pain free at 1 year postoperatively. Subsequent reports have shown similar results in adolescent patients.[18–20] Miyamoto and colleagues[20] first reported their results of this procedure in 4 adolescent female patients with late-stage disease, all of whom showed healing of the osteochondral plug and normal or near-normal chondral surface of the metatarsal head at second-look arthroscopy 1 year postoperatively. A follow-up series published in 2016 monitored the progress of 13 patients, all female, with an age range of 10 to 38 years, at a minimum of 5 years postoperatively.[19] Statistically and clinically significant improvements in American Orthopaedic Foot and Ankle Score (AOFAS) and visual analogue scale scores were noted in all patients. All of the osteochondral plugs incorporated, no patients showed progressive degenerative changes on radiographs at 2 years postoperatively, and select patients who underwent MRI at 5 years postoperatively showed normal contour of the articular surface. Although results of this technique are promising for late-stage disease, it is difficult to extrapolate the reported success beyond the adolescent population.

Metatarsal osteotomies
From the early reports on surgical treatment of Freiberg disease, metatarsal osteotomies have been used with good success, typically in combination with joint debridement. Osteotomies are generally divided into 2 options: dorsal closing-wedge osteotomies (either intra-articular or extra-articular) to reorient the preserved plantar cartilage and improve the articulation of the MTP joint (**Fig. 3**), and shortening osteotomies that decompress the metatarsal head and MTP joint. Although the more

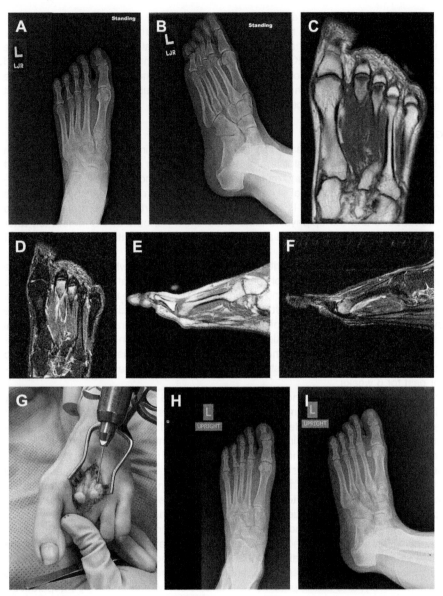

Fig. 2. This female patient in her mid-20s presented with chronic pain at both the second and third MTP joints. Imaging studies did not reveal significant collapse of the metatarsal heads (*A*, *B*) but MRI confirmed the presence of Smillie stage I disease (*C–F*). The patient failed 6 months of conservative management and underwent debridement of the second and third MTP joints with retrograde drilling into the metatarsal heads (*G*). At 1 year postoperatively, there has been no collapse or evidence of progressive degenerative changes at the metatarsal heads (*H*, *I*) and the patient remains pain free.

proximal osteotomies are typically stabilized with a small fragment plate and/or screws,[21,22] osteotomies at the metatarsal neck or head are commonly secured with Kirschner wires or sutures.[3,23–29] Cerclage wire has also been used with successful healing at the osteotomy site but with increased risk of extensor tendonitis and

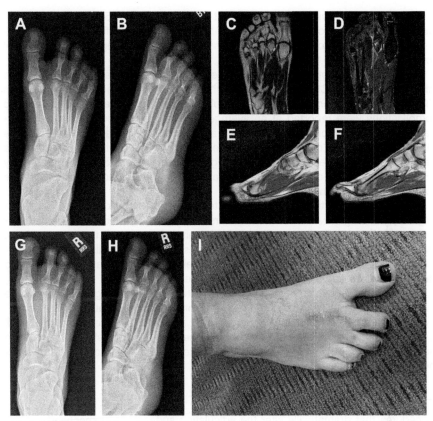

Fig. 3. This 29-year-old female patient presented with pain and swelling at the second MTP joint. Radiographic evaluation showed Smillie stage II disease with asymmetric collapse of the dorsal and lateral metatarsal head (*A–F*). The patient eventually required joint debridement with an intra-articular dorsal and lateral wedge osteotomy. The osteotomy was secured with absorbable suture. At 6 months postoperatively, the osteotomy has healed (*G, H*) and the patient has returned to activity pain free without residual elevation of the toe (*I*).

dorsal soft tissue irritation.[26,27] Lee and colleagues[30] used bioabsorbable pins to secure an intra-articular dorsal closing-wedge osteotomy with successful healing, although the cost and need for possible multiple pins limits enthusiasm for this fixation method.

The dorsiflexion osteotomy was first described by Gauthier and Elbaz[3] in 1979. The investigators used an intra-articular osteotomy at the site of the chondral injury, removing the diseased cartilage and subchondral bone and reorienting the plantar cartilage into the central joint. Symptoms improved in all but 1 of the 53 cases in the series. Kinnard and Lirette[26,27] also endorsed use of an intra-articular osteotomy with excellent results in 15 patients at an average of 50 months of follow-up. The investigators noted no cases of transfer metatarsalgia and observed that enough viable plantar cartilage and bone was present even in severe cases of Freiberg disease to warrant a joint-sparing procedure. In 2016, Pereira and colleagues[29] provided the longest follow-up of any case report for the treatment of Freiberg disease. Twenty patients with Smillie stage II to IV disease underwent an osteotomy as described by

Gauthier and Elbaz,[3] with mean follow-up of 23.4 years (range, 15–32 years). No complications with the procedure were noted. All patients were satisfied with the procedure and average postoperative AOFAS lesser metatarsophalangeal-interphalangeal score was 96.8 (range, 91–100).

Extra-articular osteotomies have also been reported with excellent short-term and mid-term outcomes. Chao and colleagues[24] noted 85% good or excellent results in 13 patients who underwent an extra-articular dorsal closing-wedge osteotomy. No complications were reported at an average follow-up of 40 months. Lee and colleagues[28] performed joint debridement and an extra-articular osteotomy in 13 patients with mean 44 months of follow-up. All patients were satisfied with the results. There were no nonunions reported and no progression of degenerative changes. Only 0.5 mm of shortening of the metatarsal head on average was noted and there were no reports of transfer metatarsalgia.

Although an intra-articular osteotomy potentially limits the risk of transfer metatarsalgia by avoiding elevation of the metatarsal head and is a technically easier procedure, fixation is more tenuous given the limited bone distal to the osteotomy. Extra-articular dorsal closing-wedge osteotomies provide more distal bone for fixation, but care must be taken not to excessively elevate the metatarsal head to avoid transfer metatarsalgia and floating toe deformities.

Smith and colleagues[22] endorsed use of a metatarsal shortening osteotomy at the level of the metatarsal neck to decompress the abnormal metatarsal head. The osteotomy was stabilized with a small fragment T plate. At a mean 4.9 years of follow-up, all but 1 of 16 patients were satisfied with the procedure, though 7 showed decreased range of motion of the MTP joint and 4 presented with dorsiflexion contractures of the toe.

Joint-Reconstructing Procedures

Procedures that dramatically alter the articulating surfaces or biomechanics of the MTP joint have been endorsed for severe Freiberg disease when there has been substantial loss of chondral tissue and congruity of the subchondral bone throughout the metatarsal head or advanced degenerative changes on both sides of the MTP joint. Care must be taken during these procedures to maintain adequate length of the toe through the MTP joint to prevent transfer metatarsalgia and dysfunction of the involved toe.

Metatarsal head resection

Although excision of the diseased metatarsal head in late-stage disease has been advocated in the past,[9] this procedure introduces an increased risk of transfer metatarsalgia, unacceptable shortening of the involved digit, and hallux valgus deformity in the case of second metatarsal Freiberg disease.[5,31,32] For these reasons, it is not recommended to perform a metatarsal head resection in isolation. These complications may be mitigated by combining a metatarsal head resection with an interpositional arthroplasty in late-stage disease.

Interpositional tissue arthroplasty

The interposition of soft tissue autograft has been used with success in patients with severe MTP degenerative changes, including those with Smillie stage IV and V disease.[8,32–38] This technique can be performed without need for large additional incisions or the increased cost of artificial implants, and preserves the length of the toe as well as an implant.[35] The dorsal MTP joint capsule,[32] extensor digitorum longus[33] or extensor digitorum brevis (EDB)[35,37,38] tendons, and free peroneus longus graft[36] have all been used as autograft to maintain joint space after thorough debridement of the MTP joint. Ozkan and colleagues[35] described a technique in which the distal attachment of the EDB tendon is preserved because the tendon is cut through a separate small incision at the musculotendinous junction. The tendon is then passed through a drill hole in the base of the proximal phalanx and then secured within the debrided MTP joint. In their retrospective review of 10 patients with Smillie grade II to IV disease, 90% good to excellent results were noted and no radiographic evidence of joint space narrowing was noted at an average of 25 months of follow-up (range, 12–36 months). Lavery and Harkless[32] used the dorsal MTP joint capsule as an interpositional graft with good to excellent results reported at an average of 3 years postoperatively in all but 1 of the 9 patients in their case series. Although all patients noted improved pain and postoperative activity levels, diminished range of motion of the MTP was observed and the thin capsular tissue was insufficient to maintain joint space. Interposition of the EDB has also been performed in conjunction with arthroscopic debridement of the MTP joint with success, although it is more technically challenging and requires specialized arthroscopic equipment.[37,38]

Allograft tendon can also be used for an interpositional arthroplasty but its widespread use is limited predominately by cost, particularly when autograft tissue is readily available at the surgical site and with minimal associated loss of function postoperatively. In later stages of Freiberg disease in which there has been progression of degenerative changes and collapse of the metatarsal head, a resurfacing arthroplasty of the metatarsal head may be considered. Acellular dermal tissue matrix tissue or other similar allograft can be secured to create a cap around the metatarsal head and allow for more normal motion at the MTP joint while maintaining some degree of joint space (**Fig. 4**). However, there is no literature currently available to guide expectations with regard to complications or the durability of this type of construct.

Osteochondral distal metatarsal allograft replacement

Bulk allograft can be used in a salvage situation when previous operative interventions, such as osteotomies or interpositional arthroplasty, have failed. Careful patient selection is paramount. This procedure may be considered for patients with metatarsal-sided degenerative changes only, and in situations in which postoperative activity demands would not be met with a metatarsal head resection. Ajis and colleagues[39] described a technique for osteochondral distal metatarsal allograft replacement with 2 patients showing avascular changes at the second metatarsal head. Both patients were satisfied with the procedure at final follow-up with complete healing noted across the graft–native bone interface and no evidence of symptomatic coronal or sagittal plane deformity. Limited degenerative changes were noted radiographically at the second MTP joint at final evaluation.

Synthetic implants

Lesser MTP joint replacement arthroplasty has been met with limited success in the literature. Silicone, ceramic, and titanium devices have been used in small case series with mixed results.[9,40–44] Numerous complications have been reported with these procedures, including prosthesis failure or loosening, synovitis, osteolysis, infection, and dysfunction of the involved toe leading to transfer metatarsalgia. For these reasons and the lack of reliable success reported in the literature, artificial joint arthroplasty cannot be recommended for treatment of late-stage Freiberg disease. The use of a synthetic cartilage (polyvinyl alcohol hydrogel) implant has generated recent support and showed success when used as an interpositional arthroplasty for the first MTP joint. The implant is not approved by the US Food and Drug Administration for use

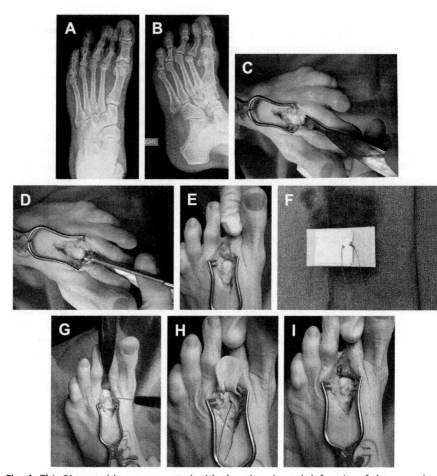

Fig. 4. This 61-year-old man presented with chronic pain and deformity of the second toe despite a previous proximal interphalangeal arthrodesis performed years before. Radiographs showed Smillie stage V disease (*A, B*). Severe collapse and degenerative changes of the metatarsal head were noted at the time of surgery with a few small loose bodies present within the joint (*C*). The patient underwent joint debridement and a resurfacing arthroplasty with acellular dermal allograft tissue. Careful debridement and reshaping of the subchondral bone was performed with 14-mm cup-and-cone reamers from a first MTP arthrodesis set (*D, E*). The dermal allograft tissue was then secured through drill holes to the plantar aspect of the metatarsal neck (*F, G*). The tissue was then carefully wrapped around the metatarsal head and trimmed to recreate a new articulating surface (*H, I*). At 6 months postoperatively, the patient noted near-complete pain relief at the second MTP joint without sagittal plane deformity.

in lesser metatarsals and although individual procedures have been performed, no literature is available at this time to support its use in treatment of Freiberg disease.

SUMMARY

Freiberg disease remains an uncommon condition but can severely affect patients' quality of life and activity, especially because most patients present with symptoms in the second or third decades of life. Conservative measures that alleviate stress on the affected metatarsal head remain the accepted first-line treatment of all stages of disease. When conservative treatment fails, operative intervention may be considered and is generally divided into joint-sparing and joint-replacing procedures. Patients with early-stage disease (Smillie I–III) are candidates for joint-sparing procedures, with most data supporting joint debridement in combination with a metatarsal osteotomy. Late-stage disease may require more aggressive debridement of the MTP joint and an arthroplasty procedure to maintain the length of the toe and limit risk of transfer metatarsalgia. Further studies are needed to support any individual procedure given the small number of patients in case series and the lack of prospective or randomized studies.

REFERENCES

1. Freiberg A. Infraction of second metatarsal bone, a typical injury. Surg Gynaecol Obstet 1914;19:191–3.
2. Cerrato RA. Freiberg's disease. Foot Ankle Clin 2011;16(4):647–58.
3. Gauthier G, Elbaz R. Freiberg's infraction: a subchondral bone fatigue fracture. A new surgical treatment. Clin Orthop Relat Res 1979;(142):93–5.
4. Hill J, Jimenez AL, Langford JH. Osteochondritis dissecans treated by joint replacement. J Am Podiatry Assoc 1979;69(9):556–61.
5. Carmont MR, Rees RJ, Blundell CM. Current concepts review: Freiberg's disease. Foot Ankle Int 2009;30(2):167–76.
6. Smillie IS. Treatment of Freiberg's infraction. Proc R Soc Med 1967;60(1):29–31.
7. Mifune Y, Matsumoto T, Mizuno T, et al. Idiopathic osteonecrosis of the second metatarsal head. Clin Imaging 2007;31(6):431–3.
8. Thompson FM, Hamilton WG. Problems of the second metatarsophalangeal joint. Orthopedics 1987;10(1):83–9.
9. Helal B, Gibb P. Freiberg's disease: a suggested pattern of management. Foot Ankle 1987;8(2):94–102.
10. Katcherian DA. Treatment of Freiberg's disease. Orthop Clin North Am 1994; 25(1):69–81.
11. Sproul J, Klaaren H, Mannarino F. Surgical treatment of Freiberg's infraction in athletes. Am J Sports Med 1993;21(3):381–4.
12. Carro LP, Golano P, Farinas O, et al. Arthroscopic Keller technique for Freiberg disease. Arthroscopy 2004;20(Suppl 2):60–3.
13. Maresca G, Adriani E, Falez F, et al. Arthroscopic treatment of bilateral Freiberg's infraction. Arthroscopy 1996;12(1):103–8.
14. Dolce MO, Osher L, McEneaney P, et al. The use of surgical core decompression as treatment for avascular necrosis of the second and third metatarsal heads. Foot 2006;17(3):162–6.
15. Freiberg AA, Freiberg RA. Core decompression as a novel treatment for early Freiberg's infraction of the second metatarsal head. Orthopedics 1995;18(12): 1177–8.
16. Lawton JH. Early surgical intervention for Freiberg's infraction: autogenous epiphysiodesis. J Foot Surg 1979;18(2):68–71.
17. Hayashi K, Ochi M, Uchio Y, et al. A new surgical technique for treating bilateral Freiberg disease. Arthroscopy 2002;18(6):660–4.
18. DeVries JG, Amiot RA, Cummings P, et al. Freiberg's infraction of the second metatarsal treated with autologous osteochondral transplantation and external fixation. J Foot Ankle Surg 2008;47(6):565–70.

19. Miyamoto W, Takao M, Miki S, et al. Midterm clinical results of osteochondral autograft transplantation for advanced stage Freiberg disease. Int Orthop 2016;40(5): 959–64.
20. Miyamoto W, Takao M, Uchio Y, et al. Late-stage Freiberg disease treated by osteochondral plug transplantation: a case series. Foot Ankle Int 2008;29(9):950–5.
21. Kim J, Choi WJ, Park YJ, et al. Modified Weil osteotomy for the treatment of Freiberg's disease. Clin Orthop Surg 2012;4(4):300–6.
22. Smith TW, Stanley D, Rowley DI. Treatment of Freiberg's disease. A new operative technique. J Bone Joint Surg Br 1991;73(1):129–30.
23. Capar B, Kutluay E, Mujde S. Dorsal closing-wedge osteotomy in the treatment of Freiberg's disease. Acta Orthop Traumatol Turc 2007;41(2):136–9 [in Turkish].
24. Chao KH, Lee CH, Lin LC. Surgery for symptomatic Freiberg's disease: extraarticular dorsal closing-wedge osteotomy in 13 patients followed for 2-4 years. Acta Orthop Scand 1999;70(5):483–6.
25. Ikoma K, Maki M, Kido M, et al. Extra-articular dorsal closing-wedge osteotomy to treat late-stage Freiberg disease using polyblend sutures: technical tips and clinical results. Int Orthop 2014;38(7):1401–5.
26. Kinnard P, Lirette R. Dorsiflexion osteotomy in Freiberg's disease. Foot Ankle 1989;9(5):226–31.
27. Kinnard P, Lirette R. Freiberg's disease and dorsiflexion osteotomy. J Bone Joint Surg Br 1991;73(5):864–5.
28. Lee HJ, Kim JW, Min WK. Operative treatment of Freiberg disease using extra-articular dorsal closing-wedge osteotomy: technical tip and clinical outcomes in 13 patients. Foot Ankle Int 2013;34(1):111–6.
29. Pereira BS, Frada T, Freitas D, et al. Long-term follow-up of dorsal wedge osteotomy for pediatric Freiberg disease. Foot Ankle Int 2016;37(1):90–5.
30. Lee SK, Chung MS, Baek GH, et al. Treatment of Freiberg disease with intra-articular dorsal wedge osteotomy and absorbable pin fixation. Foot Ankle Int 2007;28(1):43–8.
31. Hoskinson J. Freiberg's disease: a review of the long-term results. Proc R Soc Med 1974;67(2):106–7.
32. Lavery LA, Harkless LB. The interpositional arthroplasty procedure in treatment of degenerative arthritis of the second metatarsophalangeal joint. J Foot Surg 1992; 31(6):590–4.
33. el-Tayeby HM. Freiberg's infraction: a new surgical procedure. J Foot Ankle Surg 1998;37(1):23–7 [discussion: 79].
34. Myerson MS, Redfern DJ. Technique tip: modification of DuVries's lesser metatarsophalangeal joint arthroplasty to improve joint mobility. Foot Ankle Int 2004; 25(4):278–9.
35. Ozkan Y, Ozturk A, Ozdemir R, et al. Interpositional arthroplasty with extensor digitorum brevis tendon in Freiberg's disease: a new surgical technique. Foot Ankle Int 2008;29(5):488–92.
36. Zgonis T, Jolly GP, Kanuck DM. Interpositional free tendon graft for lesser metatarsophalangeal joint arthropathy. J Foot Ankle Surg 2005;44(6):490–2.
37. Lui TH. Arthroscopic interpositional arthroplasty for Freiberg's disease. Knee Surg Sports Traumatol Arthrosc 2007;15(5):555–9.
38. Lui TH. Arthroscopic interpositional arthroplasty of the second metatarsophalangeal joint. Arthrosc Tech 2016;5(6):e1333–8.
39. Ajis A, Seybold JD, Myerson MS. Osteochondral distal metatarsal allograft reconstruction: a case series and surgical technique. Foot Ankle Int 2013;34(8): 1158–67.

40. Cracchiolo A 3rd, Kitaoka HB, Leventen EO. Silicone implant arthroplasty for second metatarsophalangeal joint disorders with and without hallux valgus deformities. Foot Ankle 1988;9(1):10–8.
41. Townshend D, Greiss M. Total ceramic arthroplasty for painful destructive disorders of the lesser metatarso-phalangeal joints. Foot 2007;17:73–5.
42. Bordelon RL. Silicone implant for Freiberg's disease. South Med J 1977;70(8):1002–4.
43. Miller ML, Lenet MD, Sherman M. Surgical treatment of Freiberg's infraction with the use of total joint replacement arthroplasty. J Foot Surg 1984;23(1):35–40.
44. Shih AT, Quint RE, Armstrong DG, et al. Treatment of Freiberg's infraction with the titanium hemi-implant. J Am Podiatr Med Assoc 2004;94(6):590–3.

Moving?

Make sure your subscription moves with you!

To notify us of your new address, find your **Clinics Account Number** (located on your mailing label above your name), and contact customer service at:

Email: journalscustomerservice-usa@elsevier.com

800-654-2452 (subscribers in the U.S. & Canada)
314-447-8871 (subscribers outside of the U.S. & Canada)

Fax number: 314-447-8029

Elsevier Health Sciences Division
Subscription Customer Service
3251 Riverport Lane
Maryland Heights, MO 63043

*To ensure uninterrupted delivery of your subscription, please notify us at least 4 weeks in advance of move.

Printed and bound by CPI Group (UK) Ltd, Croydon, CR0 4YY

08/05/2025

01864709-0003